Dual Source CT Imaging
Asian Adaptation

Philipp Lengsfeld, PhD
Christoph Panknin, MS
Vivek Verma, MD

This project was supported by

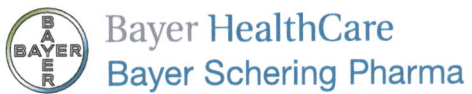

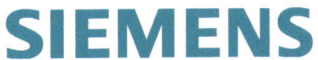

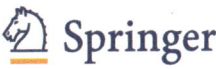

Philipp Lengsfeld, PhD
Bayer Schering Pharma AG
GMA Diagnostic Imaging
Müllerstr. 178
D-13353 Berlin, Germany

Vivek Verma, MD
63 Chulia Street
OCBC Centre East, 14th floor
Singapore 049514, Singapore

Christoph Panknin, MS
Siemens Computed Tomography, Asia Pacific
Siemens Pte Ltd, the Siemens Center, 13th Floor
60 MacPherson Road, Singapore 348615, Singapore

ISBN 978-3-642-15133-0
Springer Medizin Verlag Berlin Heidelberg New York

Bibliografische Information der Deutschen Bibliothek
The Deutsche Bibliothek lists this publication in Deutsche
Nationalbibliographie; detailed bibliographic data is
available in the internet at http://dnb.ddb.de.

Springer Medizin
Springer-Verlag GmbH
Ein Unternehmen von Springer Science+Business Media

springer.com
© Springer Medizin Verlag Berlin Heidelberg 2010

SPIN 80020856

Design and Typesetting:
A.UND.W – Agentur für Kommunikation, Berlin
Printing: Stürtz, Wüzburg

18/5138 – 5 4 3 2 1 0

Content

Dear Colleagues

It is our great pleasure to present to you the Asian adaptation of the Dual Source CT (DSCT) imaging protocol book. The original book with its case reports and protocols was compiled in 2008, providing a comprehensive source of scan and contrast protocols for all important indications for the first DSCT scanner, the Somatom Definition [1]. The book presented here is a compilation of cases and protocols especially tailored for the Asian population. The underlying rationale is that the Asian population has some significant differences (e.g. average weight of the patients) compared to the Western patient population studied for the original book, necessitating a protocol adaptation to fully utilize the potential of the DSCT technology in Asia.

The focus has been on optimizing both the scan and the contrast protocols, as the contrast media delivery has become an increasingly critical element of the contrast-enhanced procedure in modern CT imaging. Radiation exposure reduction was achieved in a number of the adapted protocols.

This project has brought together nine Asian institutions (four from China and Korea, respectively, and one site from Singapore). The protocols and cases have been jointly discussed and consolidated at two full-day workshops.

This Asian adaptation book is another outcome of the partnership of Siemens AG and Bayer Schering Pharma AG in the field of CT imaging. We hope that the recommendations in this book will go a long way in benefiting scores of patients who undergo CT scanning in this part of the world.

Yours sincerely,

Philipp Lengsfeld, PhD
Vivek Verma, MD   Christoph Panknin, MS
Bayer Schering Pharma AG   Siemens AG

[1] Seidensticker, Hofmann (Eds), Dual Source CT Imaging, Springer, 2008

DSCT Technology / Contrast Medium

Dual Source CT Technology

Bernhard Schmidt
Christiane Koch
Thomas Flohr

Siemens AG
Medical Solutions
Computed Tomography
Siemensstr. 1
D-91301 Forchheim, Germany

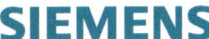

Dual Source CT Technology

The introduction of spiral CT in the early 1990s marked one of the important steps in the evolution of CT-imaging techniques.[1,2] The technology allowed clinicians for the first time to acquire volume data without the risk of mis- or double-registration. It also enabled the reconstruction of images at any position along the patient's length axis as well as reconstructions of overlapping images to improve the longitudinal resolution. Furthermore, spiral acquisition reduced scan times significantly as the patient moved continuously through the gantry rather than step-by-step (step and shoot mode).

Despite these improvements, single-slice spiral CT used in daily clinical routine presented many limitations. Because of the small detector coverage, spiral CT was only able to achieve a desired isotropic resolution (i.e. equal resolution in all three spatial axes) for very limited scan ranges.[3] For longer scans (e.g. chest examinations), the spatial resolution along the patient's length axis had to be significantly compromised. The introduction of multi-detector row computed tomography (MDCT) in 1998 solved some of these issues. Larger anatomical volumes could be acquired with a single acquisition. The first generation of MDCT systems offered simultaneous acquisition of 4 slices at a rotation time of 0.5 s, which provided considerably improved scan speed and longitudinal resolution as well as better utilization of the available x-ray power.[4–6] In addition to significantly reducing acquisition time for a variety of clinical protocols, MDCT also made longer scan ranges with substantially reduced slice width feasible, which is essential, for example, in CT angiography (CTA) of the lower extremities.[7] MDCT also expanded into areas previously considered beyond the scope of 3rd generation CT scanners using mechanical rotation of x-ray tube and detector, such as CTA of the coronary arteries with the addition of ECG gating capability.[8,9]

Despite these promising improvements, clinical challenges and limitations remained for 4-slice CT systems. True isotropic resolution for routine applications had not yet been achieved for many applications such as CTA of the chest.[7] Stents or severely calcified arteries constituted a diagnostic dilemma for ECG-gated coronary CTA, mainly due to partial volume artifacts resulting from insufficient longitudinal resolution, and limited temporal resolution made reliable imaging of patients with higher heart rates impossible.[10]

The introduction of 16-slice CT scanners finally enabled routine acquisitions with isotropic sub-millimeter spatial resolution.[11,12] This technology also opened up other new possibilities such as the diagnosis of an acute ischemic stroke by assessing the status of the vessels supplying the brain and

Dual Source CT Technology

the location of the intracranial occlusion in the same CTA examination. The higher detector coverage again improved the diagnosis of central and peripheral pulmonary embolisms, even in patients with limited ability to cooperate.[13, 14] ECG-gated cardiac scanning was enhanced by both improved temporal resolution as a result of gantry rotation times as low as 0.375 s and improved spatial resolution.[15, 16]

The generation of 64-slice CT systems was introduced in 2004. This technology relies on new scanner concepts, and two different concepts were launched on the market.

The "volume concept" pursued by GE, Philips and Toshiba aims to further increase the volume coverage speed by using 64 detector rows instead of 16 without changing the physical parameters of the scanner from the 16-slice version.

The "resolution concept" pursued by Siemens uses 32 physical detector rows in combination with "double z-sampling" – a refined z-sampling technique enabled by periodically moving the focal point in the z-direction, to simultaneously acquire 64 overlapping slices. The objective is to increase the longitudinal resolution and reduce spiral artifacts independent of pitch (see also Figure 1).[17, 18]

CTA examinations with sub-mm resolution in the pure arterial phase are possible with 64-slice CT systems, even for extended anatomical ranges. The entire thorax (350 mm) can be scanned with sub-mm resolution in about 6 s, facilitating emergency scans, for example, to check for acute pulmonary embolism. A whole-body CTA with 1500 mm scan range takes approximately the same scan time that is required for a 16-slice scanner but with a considerably improved longitudinal resolution. Overall, the improvements in spatial and temporal resolution afforded by 64-slice CT systems lead to better quantification and tracking of disease processes such as relative stenosis, perfusion and pulsatility.[19] The improved temporal resolution that results from gantry rotation times as low as 0.33 s increases the robustness of ECG-gated scanning at higher heart rates. This facilitates the successful integration of CT coronary angiography into routine clinical algorithms, although higher heart rates can still be problematic.[20, 21]

Clinical experience with 64-slice CT systems indicates that many of the issues of previous scanner generations have been solved. Scan time – one of the driving factors in the past to increase CT detector coverage – is no longer an issue in 64-slice CT systems. In fact, the table feed has to be reduced in many cases to avoid outrunning the contrast bolus (e.g. in run-offs). Nevertheless, some of the challenges in clinical routine still exist. For example, examining obese patients remains an issue because of the limited tube power. In these cases, the patient can either not be examined at all or dedicated acquisition protocols with compromised scan speed have to be used. In addition, although cardiac CT imaging has become clinical routine, image quality is often compromised by motion artifacts in patients with higher heart rates. But higher temporal resolution would generally reduce blooming artifacts caused by stents or calcifications and residual motion even at lower heart rates. Using refined algorithms such as "multi-segment reconstruction" techniques theoretically allow the improvement of temporal resolution. However, the temporal resolution can only be increased as desired at certain heart rates (see Figure 2). Some "sweet spots" exist in principle; however, it is impossible in clinical routine to somehow adjust and maintain a patient's heart rate to achieve optimal temporal resolution. Furthermore, multi-segment reconstructions rely on data consistency from two subsequent heart beats. Any inconsistencies will lead to blurred artifacts in the images, as data from two different heart beats are mixed for the reconstruction. Because the use of multi-segment reconstruction techniques shows limited clinical stability, beta blockers are routinely and widely used to decrease the heart rate to overcome the lack of temporal resolution.[22]

To solve the clinical constraints of 64-slice CT systems, Siemens Medical Solutions introduced a Dual Source CT (DSCT) system – the SOMATOM Definition – in 2005. This CT system is equipped with two x-ray tubes and two corresponding detectors. The two acquisition systems are mounted onto a rotating gantry with a 90° angular offset (see Figure 3).[23] One detector covers the entire scan field of view (about 50 cm in diameter), while the other is restricted to a smaller, central field of view. Both detectors are capable of acquiring 64 overlapping 0.6 mm slices by means of double z-sampling (z-flying focal point technology). The gantry rotation time is 0.33 s. Each of the two x-ray tubes provides up to 80 kW peak power.

DSCT provides temporal resolutions that are one quarter of the gantry rotation time, independent of the patient's heart rate. DSCT scanners also show promising potential for general radiology applications, such as the use of dose accumulation to examine obese patients, or the use of Dual Energy acquisitions. The potential applications of Dual Energy CT include tissue characterization, local blood volume quantification in contrast-enhanced scans and iodine/calcium separation enabling, for example, the automatic removal of bone from CTA examinations.

Dual Source CT Technology

Cardiac imaging

The key benefit of DSCT for cardiac scanning and coronary CT angiography is the improved temporal resolution. In a DSCT scanner, the half-scan sinogram in parallel geometry needed for an ECG-controlled image reconstruction can be split into two quarter scan sinograms, which are simultaneously acquired by the two acquisition systems in the same relative phase of the patient's cardiac cycle and at the same anatomical level due to the 90° angle between both detectors. With this approach, a constant temporal resolution equivalent to one quarter of the gantry rotation time $t_{rot}/4$ is achieved in a centered region of the scan field of view. For $t_{rot} = 0.33$ s, the temporal resolution is $t_{rot}/4 = 83$ ms, independent of the patient's heart rate (see Figure 2). Figure 4 shows a clinical example illustrating the performance of DSCT for ECG-gated coronary CTA. Going from a single-segment reconstruction to a two- or multi-segment reconstruction only slightly improves the quality of the images. However, the temporal resolution

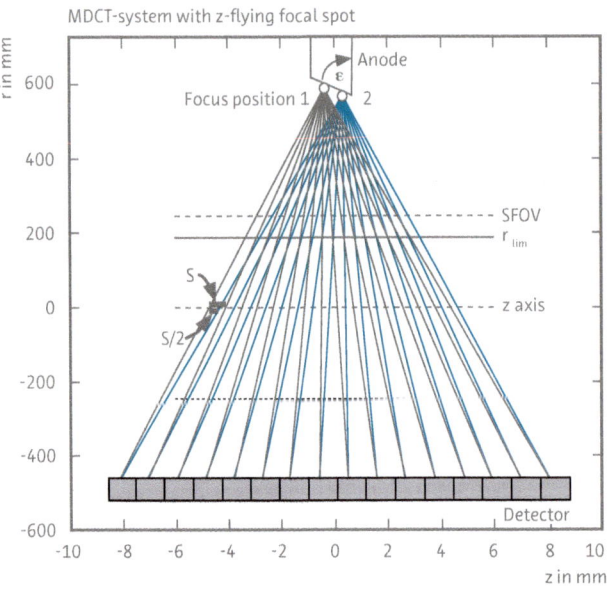

[Figure 1] Schematic illustration of improved z-sampling with the z-flying focal spot technique. Two subsequent M-slice readings are shifted by half a collimated slice width at iso-center and can be interleaved to one 2M-slice projection. Improved z-sampling is not only achieved at iso-center, but maintained in a wide range of the scan field of view (SFOV).

increase to 83 ms adds significant diagnostic value. Several clinical studies validated this information and have demonstrated that DSCT offers a very robust diagnostic image quality regardless of the heart rate.[24–27] The use of two x-ray tubes for image acquisition immediately brings up the question of patient dose, because one might assume that dose increases by a factor of two. However, the SOMATOM Definition features additional mechanisms and technical improvements that enable you to reduce the dose even below that of Single Source CT (see also Figure 5):[28]

· Additional filter: An optimized cardiac bowtie filter – widely used in CT systems – prevents unnecessary exposure outside the central heart region. The cardiac bowtie filter is dedicated and optimized for heart examinations, and it reduces the intensity outside the area of the heart even more than regular bowtie filters.

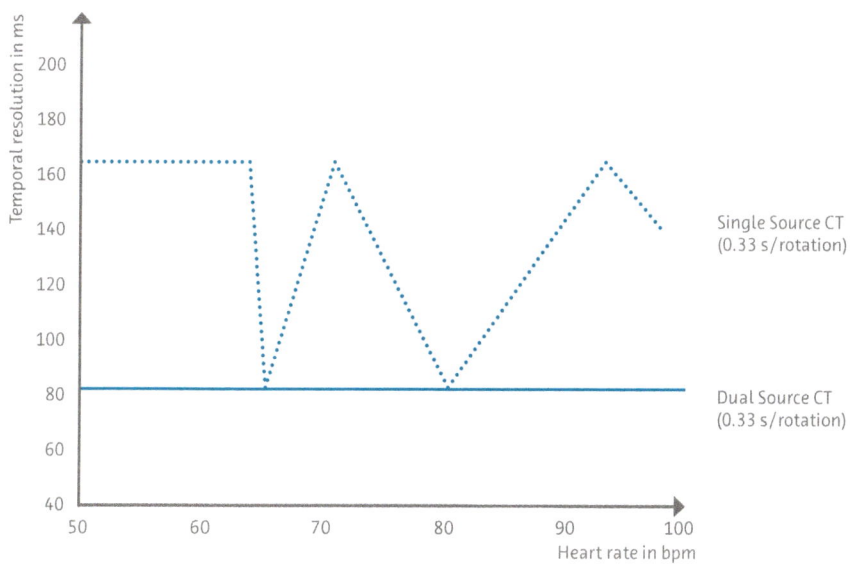

[Figure 2] Comparison of the temporal resolution of Single and Dual Source CT systems: Multi-segment reconstruction technique in the case of the Single Source systems leads to a strong dependency of the temporal resolution from the heart rate.

Dual Source CT Technology

· Pitch adaptation: Single-segment reconstruction at all heart rates enables efficient adaptation of the table feed: In Single Source CT, the only way to increase temporal resolution – which is particularly useful for patients with high heart rates – is by using the multi-segment reconstruction technique. Unfortunately, this technique requires the use of a comparatively small pitch during acquisition, resulting in longer scan times and higher radiation exposure. Conversely (and beneficially), the temporal resolution in DSCT is already in the desired range of under 100 ms in single-segment reconstruction, which make multi-segment reconstructions obsolete. Therefore, the scanning pitch can be adapted to the patient's heart rate in DSCT while it cannot in Single Source CT. The pitch increase for higher heart rates significantly reduces patient dose. It is important to note that image noise in cardiac CT is determined by the tube current product per rotation, as about 180 degrees of the complete acquisition is used to generate one image. Assuming the tube current time product (mAs)

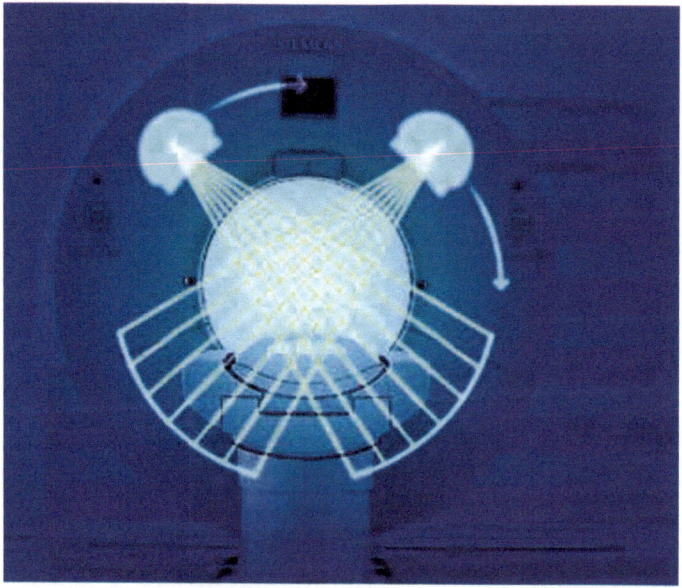

[Figure 3] Schematic illustration of a Dual Source CT (DSCT) system using two tubes and two corresponding detectors offset by 90°. This type of scanner provides temporal resolution equivalent to one quarter of the gantry rotation time for ECG-controlled cardiac CT, independent of the patient's heart rate. Both tubes can also run at different tube voltages for Dual Energy purposes.

does not change, higher pitch values will not lead to increased noise. This is true for both Single and Dual Source CT systems.

The behavior is different from conventional scanning: image noise changes with the pitch at a given mAs level. Smaller pitch values lead to less image noise than higher pitch values as all data acquired at a certain z-position contribute to the reconstructed image at that z-position.

To avoid this unwanted behavior in conventional scans, the operator specifies the "effective mAs" (mAs/pitch). Because the operator does not increase the pitch for cases of higher heart rates in Single Source cardiac CT examinations, but always uses the same small pitch level independent of the heart rate in order to be capable of multi-segment reconstructions, it was convenient for an operator to enter well-known "effective mAs" values used in regular scan mode.

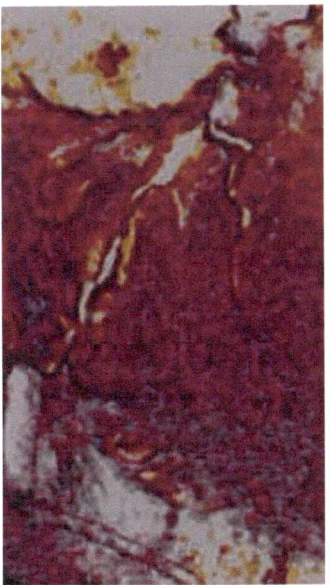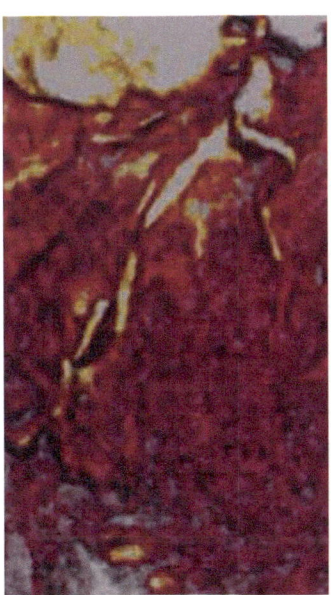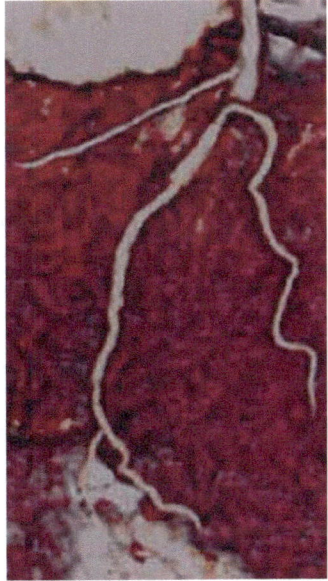

[Figure 4] Various reconstruction technique comparisons of a patient with a heart rate ranging from 86 to 122 bpm. The improvement in temporal resolution from a single- to multi-segment reconstruction only leads to insignificant improvement in image quality. The Dual Source CT reconstruction with a temporal resolution of 83 ms independent of the heart rate leads to a significant improvement in image quality. Courtesy of University Hospital of Munich-Grosshadern/Munich, Germany.

Dual Source CT Technology

The fixed pitch value established a constant relationship between "effective mAs" and the noise determining "mAs/rotation". However, the concept of "effective mAs" is not useful in DSCT systems because the pitch is adapted to the patient's heart rate. Moreover, because of this and how "effective mAs" are defined, the pitch would impact image noise. To eliminate this dependency in DSCT systems, an operator can specify "mAs per rotation". The image quality is then independent of pitch and heart rate. To provide the user control over patient dose, $CTDI_{vol}$ is displayed, which assesses the impact of pitch on patient dose.

· Optimized ECG-pulsing: New ECG-pulsing enables the reduction of exposure even in the presence of arrhythmia. It is one of the most efficient methods for dose reduction in cardiac CT. A high tube current is only used for those phases of the cardiac cycle which are required for morphology. It is

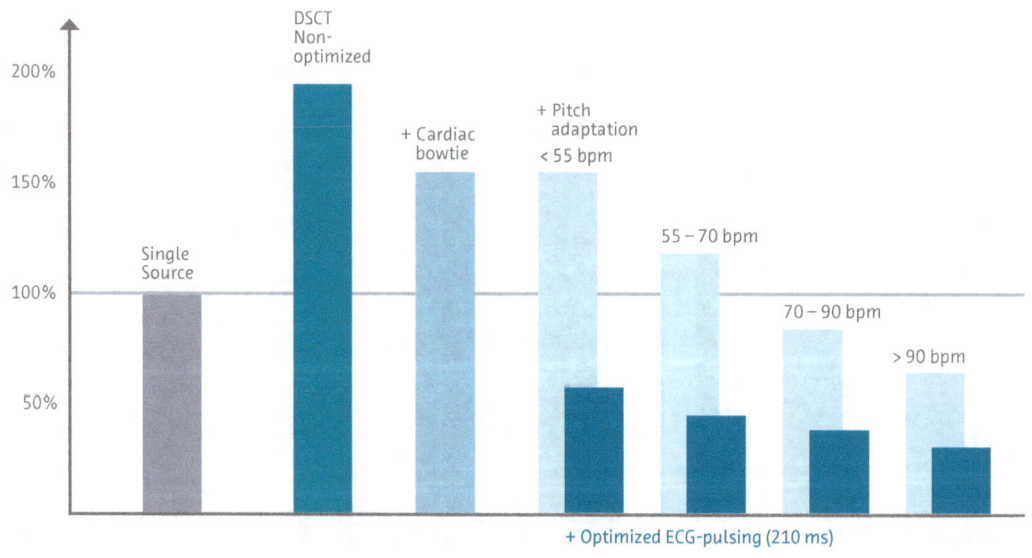

[Figure 5] Several technical improvements help to reduce patient dose in DSCT even below the level of Single Source cardiac CT.[28]

reduced for the rest of the heart cycle. These images are noisier, but they still provide diagnostic information for functional analysis. The minimum window for ECG-pulsing is determined by the time it takes to acquire 180 degrees of data. In Single Source CT, the pulsing window is about half of the rotation time; in Dual Source CT, the desired data is acquired after the gantry rotates 90 degrees. As a result, the pulsing window can be much smaller. Because different heart rates require different reconstruction time points, the plateau of full tube power should be adapted to the patient's heart rate to maximum dose savings but still be able to obtain full image quality in the data needed for a morphological diagnosis (see Table 1).

In addition to the width of the pulsing window, the level of the low dose plateau can also be used for a further dose reduction. Normally, tube current is reduced down to 20% of the nominal tube current

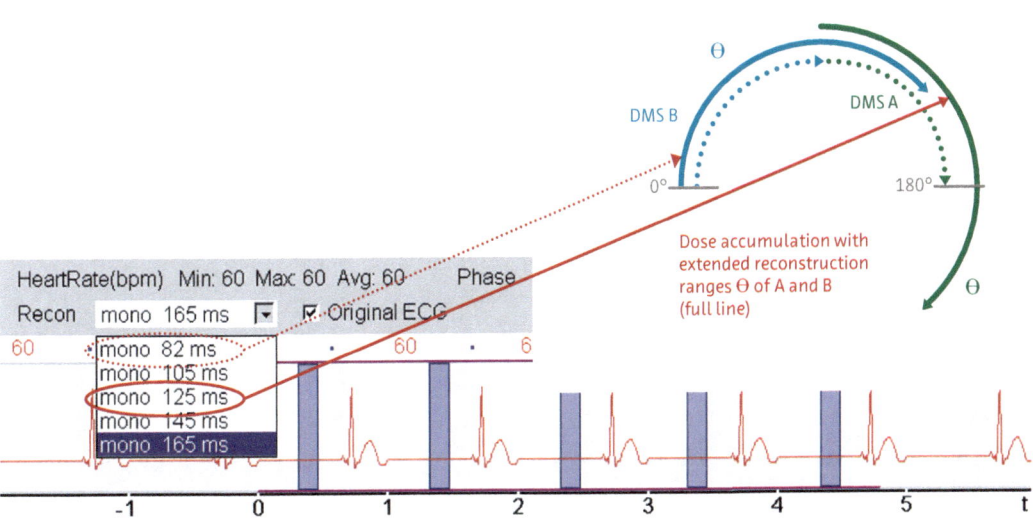

[Figure 6] Cardiac obese scanning: To further reduce image noise in cardiac scanning, temporal resolution of reconstructed images can be lowered in DSCT down to the level of a Single Source CT. Noise reduction up to a factor of $1/\sqrt{2}$ can be achieved.

Dual Source CT Technology

in the low plateau phase. The MinDose™ pulsing mode can be applied to reduce the dose even further, down to 4%. We must note that this mode does not allow the reconstruction of diagnostic data during the reduced plateau phase.

Obese imaging and cardiac obese imaging

DSCT provides powerful applications for general radiology applications as well. If both acquisition systems are simultaneously used in a standard spiral or sequential acquisition mode, an x-ray peak power of up to 160 kW is available. These power reserves are not only beneficial for the examination of morbidly obese patients, whose number is dramatically growing in western societies, but also to maintain an adequate x-ray photon flux for standard protocols when a high volume coverage speed is necessary. With Single Source CT systems, high mAs-values can only be achieved by reducing the pitch or using a slower rotation time. However, this leads to compromises in scan speed, which is sometimes unwanted or unacceptable, or at least it requires a significant change of the contrast injection protocol.

Compromising scan speed is not necessary in a DSCT system because the second tube simply adds the required power. Furthermore, the enormous tube current reserves can be used for dose reduction in contrast-enhanced examinations. The use of a lower tube voltage leads to a higher contrast of iodine. A better signal-to-noise ratio can be achieved at a lower dose level when a lower tube voltage is used. In the past, lowering of tube voltage was often not possible simply because a single x-ray tube could not provide the required tube current. The limitations of Single Source CT systems are overcome by the ability to double the mAs with a second tube.

Excessive noise when imaging obese patients is not only an issue in conventional scanning, but also in cardiac scanning, especially since reducing the pitch does not lead to less image noise in cardiac examinations. If the tube limit is reached, the only way to reduce noise in cardiac imaging is to compromise temporal resolution and collect more x-ray photons. Single Source CT systems are not

Heart Rate in bpm	Pulsing Window in %
< 60	70–70
60–80	55–80
> 80	40–80

[Table 1] In order to achieve optimal diagnostic results in coronary CTA imaging, the ECG-pulsing window should be adapted to the heart rate of the patient.

capable of this since a temporal resolution of 300 to 400 ms is not acceptable for coronary imaging. Applying the same principle to DSCT, the temporal resolution ends up in the range of about 165 ms (see Figure 6), which is still acceptable. In cardiac obese reconstruction, the temporal resolution is equal to a single-segment reconstruction of a Single Source CT. In fact, the SOMATOM Definition leaves it up to the operator to choose the reconstruction type after the examination using the same raw data, which means no additional exposure for the patient. Therefore, he or she can choose whether a regular reconstruction should be performed with a temporal resolution of 83 ms, or a dedicated "cardiac obese" reconstruction, which ends up with a temporal resolution of 165 ms but a noise level reduced by a factor of $1/\sqrt{2}$.

Dual Energy imaging

In cardiac and obese examinations, both tubes are operated with the same tube. However, both x-ray tubes can also be operated at different kV- and mAs-settings, allowing the acquisition of Dual Energy data. While Dual Energy CT was already evaluated 20 years ago, the technical limitations of the CT scanners at the time prevented the development of routine clinical applications.[29, 30] The biggest constraint was that the dose in the low voltage data was much less than in the high voltage data, since only the tube voltage was switched without adapting the tube current. Therefore, the noise level in the low voltage data was significantly higher, which finally hampered and limited the use of Dual Energy applications at that time.

With a DSCT system, Dual Energy data can be acquired nearly simultaneously in spiral mode with sub-second scan times. The ability to overcome data registration problems should prove beneficial to clinicians. Additionally, the limitations of Dual Energy from the 1980s are overcome by the utilization of two independent tube/detector systems. Noise and dose level can be adjusted independently; therefore, the same noise and dose level in both systems can be achieved by simply using a higher tube current on the low voltage system. Clinical routines have demonstrated that a tube current ratio of about 1:4 for 140kV/80kV is optimal. Depending on the Dual Energy application and the anatomical area, different collimations can be used for data acquisition similar to conventional scanning. The 64 x 0.6 mm mode is preferred for high coverage and resolution. Thinner or dedicated collimations are indicated for quantitative measurements that demand high-precision CT numbers. One of the biggest concerns is the limited field of view of the B detector (see Figure 3) because data are only acquired by the B system inside this area and as a result Dual Energy can only be performed

Dual Source CT Technology

in this area. Surprisingly, mostly all of the relevant tissue is within this inner field of view. Of course, proper positioning of the patient and the region of interest is a prerequisite. This can be done easily with the use of two topograms prior to scanning: lateral and p.a.

The use of Dual Energy CT data adds functional information to the morphological information based on x-ray attenuation coefficients that is usually obtained in a CT examination while increasing dose typically by no more than 10–30%. A potential application for Spiral Dual Energy CT is the separation of bones and iodine-filled vessels in CT angiographic examinations even in complicated anatomical situations, such as the skull base and the circle of Willis. The bones can be automatically removed, leaving only the vessels in the resultant images. The CT value of iodine increases much greater than bone or calcium with decreasing x-ray tube voltage, which is the basis for iodine-bone separation

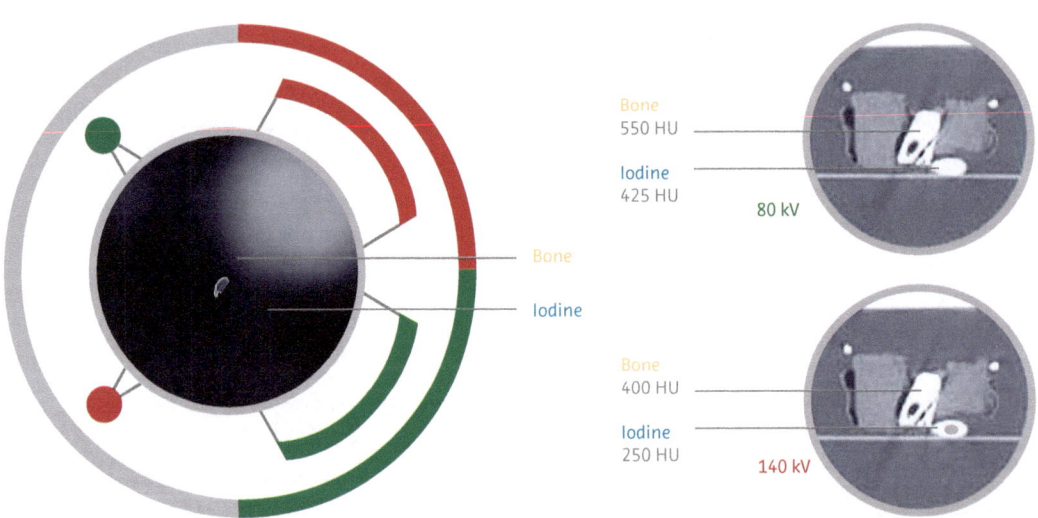

[Figure 7] Schematic illustration of the principle of Dual Energy imaging with a DSCT system. Although both tube/detector systems are mouthed with an angle of 90 degrees, images at low and high voltage are acquired simultaneously. A specimen with bony structures and tubes filled with iodine are scanned with both energy levels simultaneously. The CT number of iodine increases from high to low voltage by about a factor of 2, whereas the CT number of bone only increases slightly. These differences in CT enhancement are used to distinguish between different chemical compositions.

using Dual Energy CT (see Figure 7). The CT values for vessels filled with iodine nearly double when going from 140 kV to 80 kV, whereas bony structures show a significantly less increase in CT values with lower tube voltage.

Another example for tissue separation is the definition of renal stone composition. Uric acid and hydroxyl apatite stones can be differentiated and thus add diagnostic information simply from differences in Dual Energy behavior. A similar principle applies to the differentiation of a vessel lumen filled with iodinated blood and calcified plaques. In addition to tissue separation, Dual Energy techniques can also be used to quantify iodine concentration in tissue.[31] This allows, for example, the visualization of perfusion defects in the parenchyma in the case of a pulmonary embolism by displaying the iodine concentration of the different areas of the lungs. Another

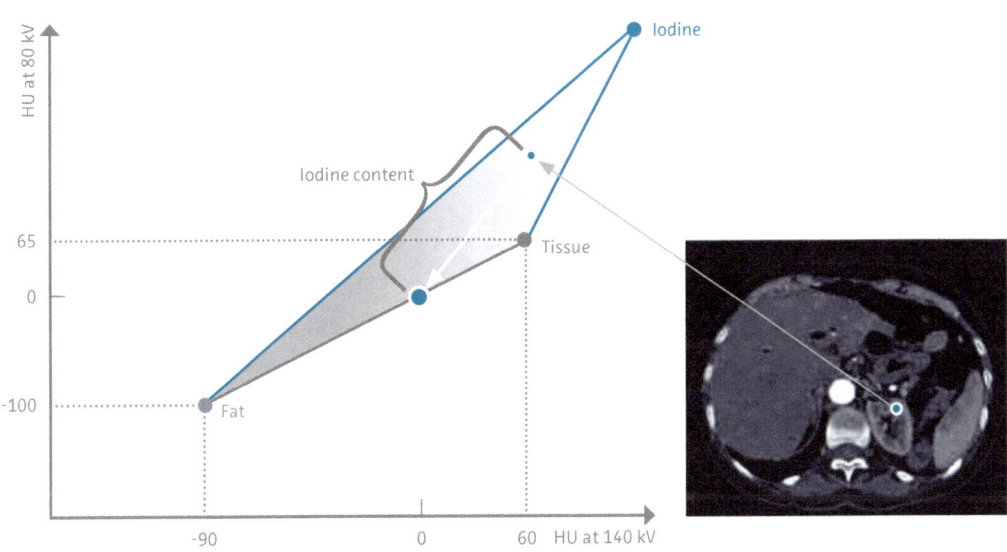

[Figure 8] Three-material decomposition: Three appropriate materials are selected depending on the anatomical location. In the case of the liver, this can be, for example, fat, tissue and iodine. After plotting all three materials into an 80 kV – 140 kV diagram, a triangle is spanned. To calculate the iodine content of ROI, CT values of this ROI at 80 kV and the 140 kV are used to determine the position of the ROI within the triangle. After projecting the point down onto the line between fat and tissue, the iodine content is determined.

Dual Source CT Technology

possible application might be the visualization of pure iodine enhancement in abdominal organs such as the kidneys. In this case, additional information about the pure enhancement might be helpful for the differential diagnosis between a hemorrhagic cyst and a renal cell carcinoma. The basic method to determine iodine concentration in tissue – and therefore also to calculate a virtual non-contrast image – is what is known as "three-material decomposition".[31] This principle is shown schematically in Figure 8. As a first step, three material/tissue types are defined that are of interest and are found in a certain anatomical area. In the liver region, this might be, for example, "soft tissue", "fat" and "iodine". Based on values from literature or clinical experience, these materials are drawn into an 80-140-kV diagram, where they span a triangle.

To evaluate a certain area of interest, the respective CT values in the 80 kV and 140 kV image are plotted into the existing diagram. Projecting this point onto the line between "fat" and "soft tissue" allows the calculation of true iodine enhancement in the region of interest. By applying this method to the whole field of view, an image showing true enhancement can be calculated. In addition to that, the image showing true enhancement can be subtracted from the weighted sum of the low and high voltage image and by doing so a "virtual" non-contrast image be calculated. Although several dedicated Dual Energy applications are already available as products, further modifications of existing and new applications are expected soon.

The evolution from sequential to spiral or from single-slice to multi-slice CT systems has revolutionized how CT systems are used in clinical routine. Clinicians all over the world are realizing and experiencing the benefits of this new, innovative technology. Although the era of Dual Source CT has just begun, DSCT systems have already provided proven results in the fields of cardiac imaging, obese imaging and Spiral Dual Energy. Dual Source CT will continue to prove the modality of choice for many other imaging procedures.

References

[1] Crawford, C. R., and K. F. King. Computed tomography scanning with simultaneous patient translation. Med Phys 1990; 17; 967-82

[2] Kalender, W. A., W. Seissler, E. Klotz, et al. Spiral volumetric CT with single-breath-hold technique, continuous transport, and continuous scanner rotation. Radiology 1990; 176; 181-3

[3] Kalender, W. A. Thin-section three-dimensional spiral CT: is isotropic imaging possible? Radiology 1995; 197; 578-80

[4] Hu, H., H. D. He, W. D. Foley, et al. Four multidetector-row helical CT: image quality and volume coverage speed. Radiology 2000; 215; 55-62

[5] Klingenbeck-Regn, K., S. Schaller, T. Flohr, et al. Subsecond multi-slice computed tomography: basics and applications. Eur J Radiol 1999; 31; 110-24

[6] McCollough, C. H., and F. E. Zink. Performance evaluation of a multi-slice CT system. Med Phys 1999; 26; 2223-30

[7] Rubin, G. D., A. J. Schmidt, L. J. Logan, et al. Multi-detector row CT angiography of lower extremity arterial inflow and runoff: initial experience. Radiology 2001; 221; 146-58

[8] Kachelriess, M., S. Ulzheimer, and W. A. Kalender. ECG-correlated image reconstruction from subsecond multi-slice spiral CT scans of the heart. Med Phys 2000; 27; 1881-902

[9] Ohnesorge, B., T. Flohr, C. Becker, et al. Cardiac imaging by means of electrocardiographically gated multisection spiral CT: initial experience. Radiology 2000; 217; 564-71

[10] Nieman, K., M. Oudkerk, B. J. Rensing, et al. Coronary angiography with multi-slice computed tomography. Lancet 2001; 357; 599-603

[11] Flohr, T., H. Bruder, K. Stierstorfer, et al. New technical developments in multislice CT, part 2: sub-millimeter 16-slice scanning and increased gantry rotation speed for cardiac imaging. Rofo 2002; 174; 1022-7

[12] Flohr, T., K. Stierstorfer, H. Bruder, et al. New technical developments in multislice CT--Part 1: Approaching isotropic resolution with sub-millimeter 16-slice scanning. Rofo 2002; 174; 839-45

[13] Remy-Jardin, M., I. Tillie-Leblond, D. Szapiro, et al. CT angiography of pulmonary embolism in patients with underlying respiratory disease: impact of multislice CT on image quality and negative predictive value. Eur Radiol 2002; 12; 1971-8

[14] Schoepf, U. J., C. R. Becker, L. K. Hofmann, et al. Multislice CT angiography. Eur Radiol 2003; 13; 1946-61

[15] Nieman, K., F. Cademartiri, P. A. Lemos, et al. Reliable noninvasive coronary angiography with fast submillimeter multislice spiral computed tomography. Circulation 2002; 106; 2051-4

[16] Ropers, D., U. Baum, K. Pohle, et al. Detection of coronary artery stenoses with thin-slice multi-detector row spiral computed tomography and multiplanar reconstruction. Circulation 2003; 107; 664-6

[17] Flohr, T., K. Stierstorfer, R. Raupach, et al. Performance evaluation of a 64-slice CT system with z-flying focal spot. Rofo 2004; 176; 1803-10

[18] Flohr, T. G., K. Stierstorfer, S. Ulzheimer, et al. Image reconstruction and image quality evaluation for a 64-slice CT scanner with z-flying focal spot. Med Phys 2005; 32; 2536-47

[19] Vrtiska, T. J., J. G. Fletcher, and C. H. McCollough. State-of-the-art imaging with 64-channel multidetector CT angiography. Perspect Vasc Surg Endovasc Ther 2005; 17; 3-8

[20] Leber, A. W., A. Knez, F. von Ziegler, et al. Quantification of obstructive and nonobstructive coronary lesions by 64-slice computed tomography: a comparative study with quantitative coronary angiography and intravascular ultrasound. J Am Coll Cardiol 2005; 46; 147-54

[21] Raff, G. L., M. J. Gallagher, W. W. O'Neill, et al. Diagnostic accuracy of noninvasive coronary angiography using 64-slice spiral computed tomography. J Am Coll Cardiol 2005; 46; 552-7

[22] Leschka, S., S. Wildermuth, T. Boehm, et al. Noninvasive coronary angiography with 64-section CT: effect of average heart rate and heart rate variability on image quality. Radiology 2006; 241; 378-85

[23] Flohr, T. G., C. H. McCollough, H. Bruder, et al. First performance evaluation of a dual-source CT (DSCT) system. Eur Radiol 2006; 16; 256-68

[24] Achenbach, S., D. Ropers, A. Kuettner, et al. Contrast-enhanced coronary artery visualization by dual-source computed tomography--initial experience. Eur J Radiol 2006; 57; 331-5

[25] Johnson, T. R., K. Nikolaou, B. J. Wintersperger, et al. Dual-source CT cardiac imaging: initial experience. Eur Radiol 2006

[26] Scheffel, H., H. Alkadhi, A. Plass, et al. Accuracy of dual-source CT coronary angiography: First experience in a high pre-test probability population without heart rate control. Eur Radiol 2006; 16; 2739-47

[27] Schertler, T., H. Scheffel, T. Frauenfelder, et al. Dual-source computed tomography in patients with acute chest pain: feasibility and image quality. Eur Radiol 2007

[28] McCollough, C. H., A. N. Primak, O. Saba, et al. Dose performance of a 64-channel dual-source CT scanner. Radiology 2007; 243; 775-84

[29] Vetter JR, Perman WH, Kalender WA, Mazess RB, Holden JE. Evaluation of a prototype dual-energy computed tomographic apparatus. II. Determination of vertebral bone mineral content. Medical Physics, 1986, 13: 340-343

[30] Kalender WA, Perman WH, Vetter JR, Klotz E. Evaluation of a prototype dual-energy computed tomographic apparatus. I. Phantom studies. Med. Phys., 1986, 13(3): 334-339

[31] Johnson, T. R., B. Krauss, M. Sedlmair, et al. Material differentiation by dual energy CT: initial experience. Eur Radiol 2007; 17; 1510-7

Ultravist®
New Perspectives with Dual Source CT

Matthias Bräutigam
Philipp Lengsfeld*
Ute Hübner-Steiner
Hubertus Pietsch

Bayer Schering Pharma AG
Research Group Diagnostic Imaging
Global Medical Affairs Diagnostic Imaging (*)
Müllerstr. 178, D-13342 Berlin, Germany

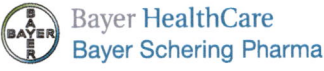
Bayer HealthCare
Bayer Schering Pharma

Ultravist®
New Perspectives with Dual Source CT

Ultravist® is a standard contrast agent in the best sense: it was introduced more than 25 years ago as one of the first products of the now dominating class of non-ionic triiodinated molecules. During these twenty-five years, millions of patients suffering from every conceivable disease, newborns, pregnant women as well as multimorbid elderly patients, patients with serious conditions such as generalized atherosclerosis, acute brain or cardiac infarctions, advanced cancer, severe cardiac insufficiency, impaired renal or hepatic function and patients of all races and living all over the world have received Ultravist® by all conceivable routes of administration. The properties of Ultravist® have been documented in hundreds of publications. It is presented in a large variety of useful concentrations and volumes (see Figure 1).

Ultravist® is a global brand, approved and used in more than 120 countries combining osmolality, viscosity and iodine in a well-balanced concentration. Currently, Ultravist® is being applied more than 10 million times a year. By mid 2010, there have been in total over 140 million applications of Ultravist® to patients.

Ultravist® – just like other non-ionic contrast agents – is a very well tolerated product which has been administered to critically ill patients at doses of more than 500 ml in adults, which is equivalent to about 150 g iodine or 300 g iopromide, the active ingredient of Ultravist®.[1–3] It may be assumed that any risks due to the administration of Ultravist® are known.[4–7] After so many years of experience and use, it is very unlikely that unexpected adverse effects will be observed.

Imaging technology determines the performance of contrast agents

As with all other x-ray contrast agents, the diagnostic capability of Ultravist® depends upon the radiological equipment used. Ever since its introduction, CT has again and again drastically changed the use of contrast media (CM). Dual Source CT is another major step in this process.

CT changed the efficacy of iodinated CM in two ways (see Figure 2a):

· Sensitivity for the detection of iodine in CT depends on the iodine concentration, whereas in standard projection x-ray procedures such as angiography the amount of iodine present along the path of the x-ray through the tissue is decisive for its detection.

Ultravist®
New Perspectives with Dual Source CT

· CT is much more sensitive to iodine than projection radiography. CT clearly visualizes iodine concentrations of 1 mg/ml in a volume of less than 0.1 ml (see Figure 2b). Projection imaging requires at least 20 mg I/ml if an object of 1 cm thickness is visualized. Angiography may serve as an example to illustrate the difference between CT and projection radiography. In spite of high contrast medium doses and very fast injection, intravenous DSA does not reliably yield clinically useful image quality because its sensitivity to iodine is too low. The contrast medium concentration in blood achieved with identical doses is fully sufficient for CT. Conversely, CTA is limited by its spatial and temporal resolution.

A very important feature is speed. The first CT scanners in the seventies took several minutes to acquire the data for a single slice. Short-lasting contrast enhancement was missing.

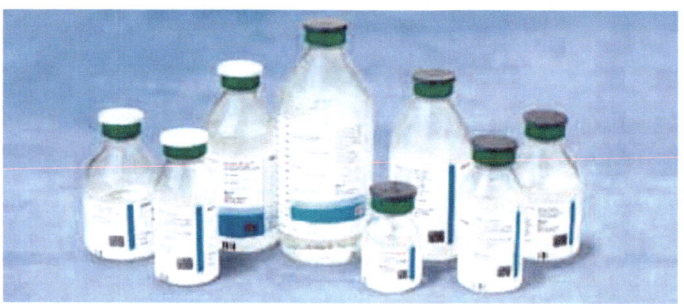
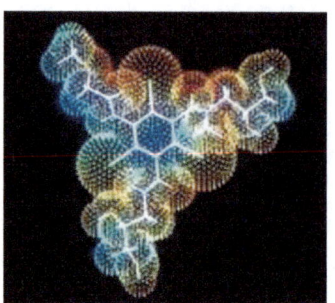

Ultravist® 370
769 mg Iopromide/ml; 370 mg I/ml
Osmolality: 770 mosm/ml
Viscosity (37°C): 10 mPa · s
Density (20°C). 1.409 g/ml

Ultravist® 300
623 mg Iopromide/ml; 300 mg I/ml
Osmolality: 590 mosm/ml
Viscosity (37°C): 4.7 mPa · s
Density (20°C): 1.328 g/ml

Iopromide
Molecular weight: 791 D
Iodine content: 48%
Size of the molecules: < 1 nm in diameter

Ultravist® 240
499 mg Iopromide/ml; 240 mg I/ml
Osmolality: 480 mosm/ml
Viscosity (37°C): 2.8 mPa · s
Density (20°C): 1.263 g/ml

Ultravist® 150
312 mg Iopromide/ml; 150 mg I/ml
Osmolality: 330 mosm/ml
Viscosity (37°C): 1.5 mPa · s
Density (20°C): 1.164 g/ml

[Figure 1] Ultravist® Technical Information.

Equally important is spatial resolution. If contrast enhancement is restricted to small lesions, it may be missed if low spatial resolution results in the display of average density values over larger volumes. High spatial resolution of moving structures can only be achieved if data acquisition is fast enough to avoid movement artifacts. Movement is critical in organs within or close to the thorax or the heart or in any other organ, tissue or structure in patients who are unable to follow the instructions of radiographers or physicians during image acquisition. The previous chapter in this book points out the dramatic progress in spatial and temporal resolution of modern CT scanners.

CT discovers the multi-talent of Ultravist®
Non-invasive angiography and the visualization of perfusion, permeability and interstitial space: Non-ionic contrast media are the current end point of a development which began about 80 years ago

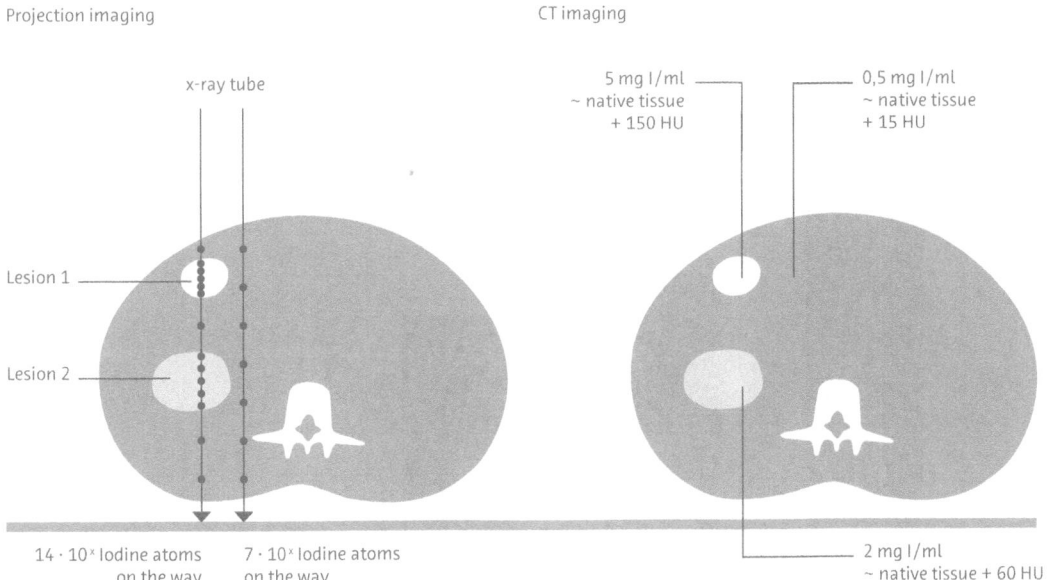

[Figure 2a] Contrast in Projection Radiography and CT.

Ultravist®
New Perspectives with Dual Source CT

with the first intravenous urographic agents. As the name says, these were iodinated contrast media aimed at visualizing the urinary tract following intravenous injection. In addition to urography, they were used from the beginning to visualize open and closed body cavities including blood vessels because they mixed with the aqueous contents of the cavities, were usually well tolerated and completely excreted within a short time. Later on it was realized that compounds belonging to the class of urographic CM did not enter cells or pass biological barriers which in practice means that they are not enterally absorbed and do not accumulate in any organs or tissues other than the kidney to a diagnostically useful extent. Because of this property, urographic CM were also called extracellular CM. Before the introduction of modern CT, urographic CM were named non-specific CM expressing the frustration of their users about the fact that they did not display structures or tissues distant from the site of injection and other than the urinary tract although they distribute

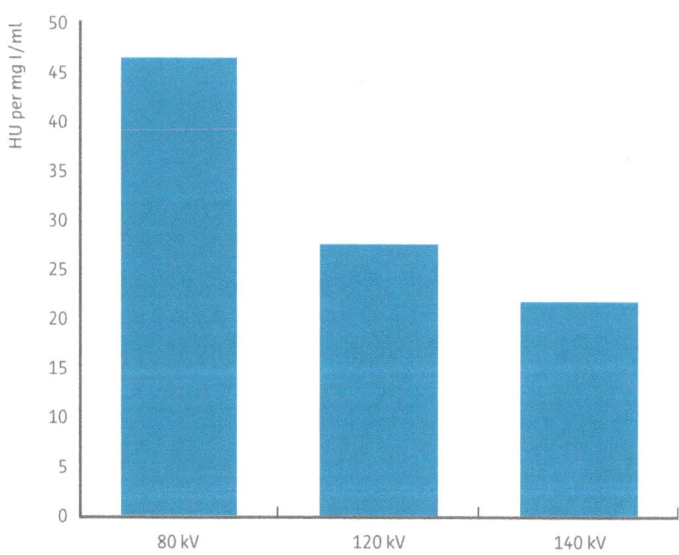

[Figure 2b] Iodine absorption (HU per mg I/ml). Probes of iodine containing solutions were investigated in a human equivalent body phantom. Measurement was performed in a Siemens Sensation 64.

throughout the body with the exception of the central nervous system to which they have no access due to the blood-brain barrier. The term 'non-specific' is misleading (see Figure 3). It is not the contrast agent which is non-specific but the way it was used due to the lack of appropriate imaging modalities. The diagnostic benefit of the extracellular CM was only slowly appreciated after the introduction of CT, with the increase in speed of data acquisition and the scanning of large volumes within a few seconds.

Urographic CM are small molecules which are unable to pass cell membranes due to their hydrophilicity. After injection, small extracellular CM molecules ideally do not interact with any body function or constituent. They diffuse through tiny pores wherever the permeability of membranes allows their passage without passing the lipid layer of a cell membrane and are carried by the blood stream to all

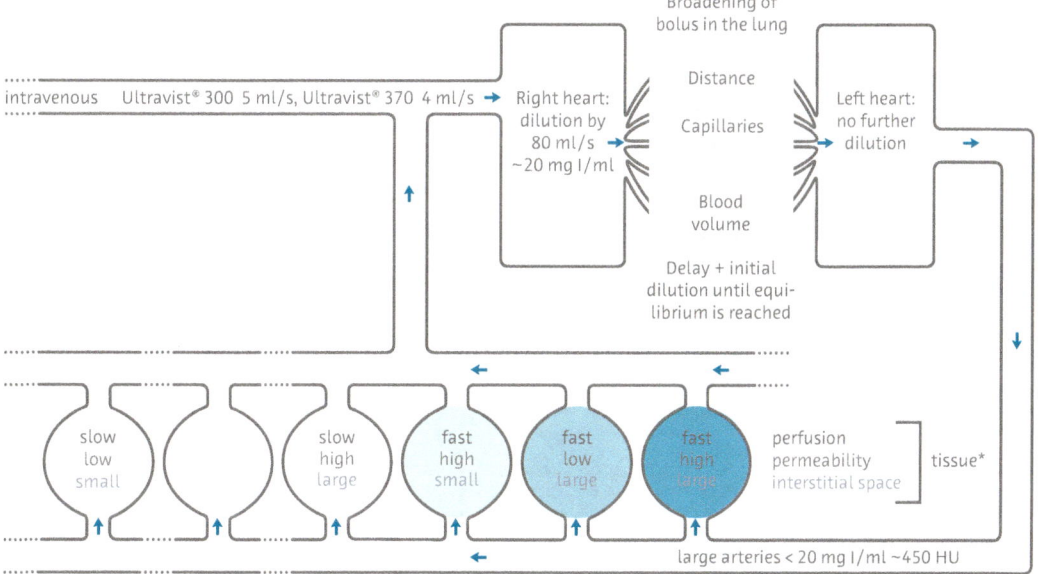

[Figure 3] Dilution and Early Pharmaco-
kinetics of Extracellular Contrast Media.

* tissue: interstitial space includes plasma volume (e.g. 5% of tissue volume, contributes about 30 HU) plus interstitial space between cells of solid tissue (e.g. 10% of tissue volume). In brain, the interstitial space is not accessible to contrast media due to the blood-brain barrier.

Ultravist®
New Perspectives with Dual Source CT

tissues, exactly reflecting blood perfusion. They are finally filtered by the glomeruli, concentrated in the renal tubules and excreted with the urine. Even if injected behind the blood-brain barrier, e.g. in myelography, elimination from the cerebrospinal fluid follows the same principles: the CM is washed out by the bulk water flow through a valve-like mechanism which allows much larger molecules to pass. Distribution and excretion are completely passive and require no additional energy except possibly concentrating the contrast agent in renal tubules.

If the extracellular CM with an iodine concentration of 300 – 370 mg I/ml is intravenously injected at a rate of 3–8 ml/s at a dose of about 1 ml/kg body weight, it is diluted by the cardiac circulation (~ 80 ml/s) and during passage through the lungs to an arterial concentration of 10 to < 20 mg I/ml, providing several hundred Hounsfield units of contrast enhancement in the arterial blood.[8] If scanning is fast enough to follow the arterial contrast agent bolus, even small arteries can be distinguished from adjacent tissue. Only after one recirculation do the dilution of the contrast medium and diffusion into the interstitial space of most tissues diminish the contrast to an extent that makes the visualization of small-caliber arteries impossible. Rapid and precisely timed scanning of large volumes is an essential precondition for CT angiography. Differentiation between calcium and iodine by Dual Energy capability further improves the quality of diagnostic information of CTA.

Although CM such as Ultravist® float passively with the bulk fluid or diffuse through tiny pores in the capillaries into the interstitial space of tissues, they provide information on the kind of tissue and important pathophysiological changes characteristic of many diseases:

Tissue perfusion
· different in different tissues
· increased in inflammation, rapidly growing tumors
· decreased in ischemia, certain tumors
· absent in cysts, infarcted or necrotic tissue

Capillary permeability
· different in different tissues
· increased in inflammation, angiogenesis, tumors
· detects disturbed blood-brain barrier

Interstitial space (including plasma volume)
· different in blood (about 55%) and tissues (about 5 – 25%)
· increased in inflammation, vascular edema, many tumors
· decreased in cellular edema

The specific distribution is, however, transient; in many cases, it can be observed only for seconds after rapid intravascular injection during the first pass of the contrast agent through the tissues and disappears after recirculation. Therefore, rapid and repeated scanning of the whole volume of interest is required to make use of the specific dynamics and early distribution pattern.

The term 'non-specific' was coined for the class of CM to which Ultravist® belongs at a time when radiographic imaging was either not capable of detecting the iodine concentrations in the interstitial space of tissues or not fast enough to image the very short period of contrast medium distribution before an equilibrium is reached, which equalizes fast and slow perfusion and diffusion into the tissue.

Contrast medium injection rate, concentration, and dose
With a few exceptions (e.g. display of blood-brain barrier disturbance), the specificity of Ultravist® following intravascular injection lasts only for seconds to a few minutes. Therefore, in many cases rapid injection is necessary to visualize pathology (see Figure 3). Since contrast depends exclusively on iodine, the injection rate has to be related to the amount of iodine injected per second (~'iodine delivery rate'). The injection rate should be as fast as possible but it is limited by the caliber of the cannula, the outflow of the vein selected for injection and the viscosity of the contrast agent. The latter may be reduced by choosing a not too high iodine concentration and by warming up the contrast medium to 37°C. Applying hand injection, the same or higher iodine delivery rates were obtained for e.g. Ultravist® 370 than for a preparation containing 400 mg I/ml.[9] Using a different catheter, Jung et al. reached slightly higher iodine delivery rates with Ultravist® 300 than with either Ultravist® 370 or Iopamidol 370.[10] The advantage of less concentrated (e.g. 300 mg I/ml) over more concentrated contrast media in respect of injection and iodine delivery rates at room temperature and at 37°C was confirmed.[11, 12] In vivo, a slightly slower intravenous injection of concentrated contrast media may be compensated or even overcompensated because a higher concentration may be maintained after dilution by a given rate of blood flow. In practice, this small difference is lost because concentrated contrast media do not mix well with blood and seem to pass the lung only slowly. Intravenous injection

Ultravist®
New Perspectives with Dual Source CT

of highly concentrated contrast media may result in lower arterial iodine concentration than the same iodine dose of a less concentrated preparation delivered in the same time.

When two iodine concentrations are compared in CTA using a fixed iodine delivery rate in both arms, no significant differences could be observed in favor of the higher concentration.[13] A sample result is presented in Figure 4. The results are in agreement with a similar study comparing Omnipaque 300 and 350 and computer simulation.[14, 15] When highly concentrated contrast media are injected at higher iodine doses than less concentrated preparations (e.g. at the same volume) or higher iodine delivery rates (i.e. same injection rate as less concentrated preparations), disadvantages of the higher viscosity may not become apparent.[16]

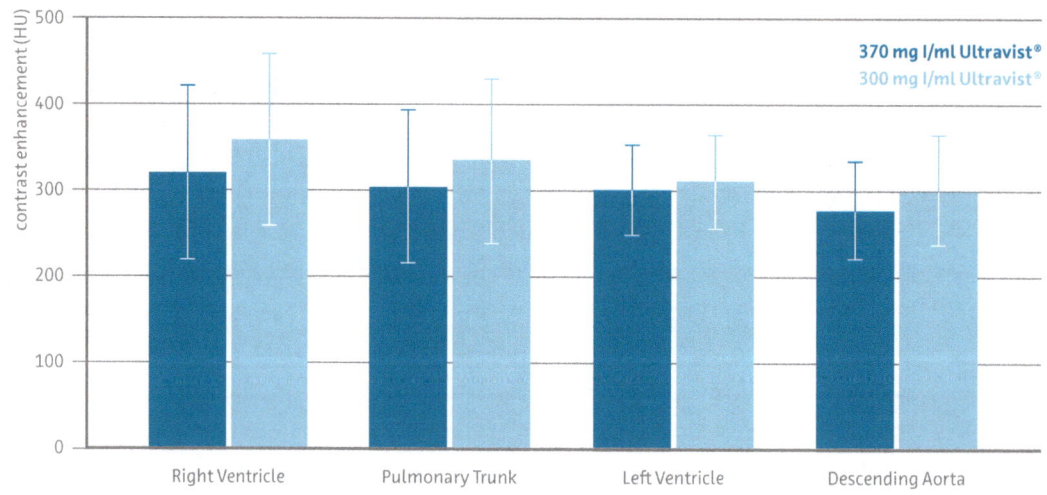

[Figure 4] Intraindividual comparison of the mean contrast enhancement in different body regions with 370 mg I/ml and 300 mg I/ml contrast media. Graphs represent mean HU±SD. The IDR in both study arms was set to 1.29 g I/s.[13]

It is obvious that high arterial blood levels can be obtained by increasing the iodine dose.[17] This is, however, the least desirable way to increase the diagnostic yield. Increased injection rate and central position of the venous catheter further increase peak iodine concentration in arterial blood. The increase of the injection rate beyond 5 or 8 ml/s does not result in a further increase in contrast.[17, 18] Dose may be fixed for a specific diagnostic problem or adjusted to body weight or lean body weight.[19] Adjustment to body weight may not be required if arterial contrast enhancement is the primary goal because the volume of the central circulation does not increase proportionally with body weight. A variety of injection protocols has been recommended for clinical routine.[20, 21] In general, choosing a suitable iodine concentration, injection rate, a saline chasing bolus, optimal timing and the fastest possible scanning technique saves contrast medium load which may better be used to obtain additional diagnostic information.

Optimizing safety
Considering the high dose and fast intravascular injection, non-ionic x-ray contrast agents belong to the least toxic compounds known. Nevertheless, a variety of unintended (e.g. feeling of warmth) or adverse effects are known and although extremely rare, a fatal idiosyncratic reaction cannot be completely excluded.

Recognizing the risk factors of individual patients and if possible reducing the risk by appropriate pre-treatment or other safety measures is the subject of numerous research articles, reviews, book chapters and recommendations of radiological and cardiological societies.[6, 7, 22] It is not the purpose of this article to provide an overview of risks, prophylaxis and treatment of contrast media reactions.

Ultravist®
New Perspectives with Dual Source CT

Renal Tolerance

In CT, contrast media are administered orally or intravenously. Recently, renal tolerance of x-ray contrast media has been disputed in patients with preexisting renal insufficiency, especially if they suffer from diabetes.[23-27] It must, however, be noticed that almost all studies reporting contrast-induced nephropathy refer to intraarterial administration. In these patients, thromboembolic complications are not rare (e.g. TIA's), and this may also contribute to deterioration of kidney function. Transient increases in serum creatinine in the patients who received contrast media meeting a certain definition of the investigators have been reported as contrast-induced nephropathy. This will necessarily include a proportion of changes due to the basic physiological and pathological fluctuation of serum creatinine as well as patients whose renal function would also have deteriorated without contrast medium exposure. Few studies were performed with intravenous injection of contrast agents at dose levels typical for CT. Among these were only two controlled studies comparing creatinine fluctuations in patients following CT with and without contrast enhancement.[28, 29] In these studies, very similar serum creatinine increases (and decreases) were observed in both groups, with and without contrast medium, pointing to the limitations of uncontrolled studies in severely ill patients. Thus, the question if, in which patient population and how frequently a clinically significant impairment of renal function occurs following intravenous administration of contrast media in CT remains unanswered.[30-32]

Even for coronary angiography with and without PCI an alleged advantage of the iso-osmolar contrast agent iodixanol regarding renal tolerance – a hypothesis generated by the 129-patients NEPHRIC study[23] – has not been confirmed in much larger studies in risk patients with various low-osmolar contrast agents including Ultravist®.[33-36] The largest randomized study to date (n = 527)[35] investigating serum creatinine changes after contrast application in renally impaired patients with diabetes undergoing coronary angiography with or without PCI has failed to detect significant differences between the iodixanol group and the low-osmolar comparator, but has shown a strong tendency against iodixanol in the 'conservative CIN rate' (serum creatinine changes in patients, where no likely non-contrast related cause was found). New preclinical work[37-39] and a large registry analysis (n > 57,000)[24] actually implicate iodixanol as being the agent with the lower renal tolerance compared to low-osmolar contrast agents. This is related to the fact that iso-osmolar, high-viscous dimers are retained longer in the kidney and are being concentrated much stronger in the kidney.[39]

Conclusion

Iodinated contrast agents are an essential component of CT. During its own development, CT helped to explore the formerly unrevealed potential of contrast media as markers of pathophysiological signs of diseases. The currently dominating and most useful type of contrast medium (urographic, extracellular marker of blood vessels, perfusion, permeability and interstitial space) was discovered in the late twenties of the last century (Uroselectan), developed further to Urografin with an improved iodine content and tolerance in the fifties, and then Ultravist® (first introduced in 1985). Ultravist® is well suited for CT with optimal concentrations and low viscosity for the fastest possible iodine delivery rate and good tolerance, which allows the injection of high single and cumulative doses. Extensive experience of 25 years and millions of applications provides the basis for a realistic assessment of the benefits and risks associated with the use of Ultravist® in the broad variety of patients referred to undergo a CT examination.

Ultravist®
New Perspectives with Dual Source CT

References

1 Rau T, Mathey D, Schofer J. High-dose tolerance of iodinated x-ray contrast media. New Developments in X-Ray and MR Angiography Symposium CIRSE, 9.9.96, Funchal, Madeira. In: Springer, Insert in Cardiovascular and Interventional Radiology 1997; 20:8-9

2 Rosovsky MA, Rusinek H, Berenstein A, et al. High-dose administration of nonionic contrast media: a retrospective review. Radiology 1996;200:119-122

3 Feldkamp T, Baumgart D, Elsner M, et al. Nephrotoxicity of iso-osmolar versus low-osmolar contrast media is equal in low risk patients. Clinical Nephrology 2006;66:322-330

4 Mortelé KJ, Oliva M-R, Ondategui S, et al. Universal use of nonionic iodinated contrast medium for CT: Evaluation of safety in a large urban teaching hospital. AJR 2005;185:31-34

5 Kopp AF, Mortelé KJ, Cho YD, Palkowitsch P, Bettmann MA, Claussen CD. Prevalence of acute reactions to iopromide: postmarketing surveillance study of 74,717 patients. Acta Radiol 2008;49:902-11

6 Morcos SK, Thomsen HS. Adverse reactions to iodinated contrast media. Eur Radiol 2001;11:1267-1275

7 Morcos SK, Thomsen HS, Webb JAW, et al. Prevention of generalized reactions to contrast media: a consensus report and guidelines. Eur Radiol 2001;11:1720-1728

8 Gmelin E, Friedrich H-J. Bolusgeometrie bei unterschiedlicher zentraler und peripherer Kontrastmittelapplikation: Studie mittels Serio-CT unter Verwendung nichtionischen Kontrastmittels. Röntgen-Bl 1985;38:219-223

9 Busch HP, Stocker KP. „Iodine delivery rate" bei der Katheterangiographie unter Druckbedingungen der manuellen Injektion. Akt Radiol 1998;8:232-235

10 Jung F, Schmitt RM, Scheller B, et al. Flussraten von Röntgenkontrastmitteln verschiedener Viskosität in 4.1-Charrière-Koronarkathetern. Z Kardiol 1996;85(8):537-542

11 Hughes PM, Bisset R. Non-ionic contrast media: a comparison of iodine delivery rates during manual injection angiography. Br J Radiol 1991;64:417-419

12 Knollmann F, Schimpf K, Felix R. Jodeinbringungsgeschwindigkeit verschieden konzentrierter Röntgenkontrastmittel bei schneller intravenöser Injektion. Fortschr Röntgenstr 2004;176:880-884

13 Behrendt FF, Mahnken AH, Stanzel S et al. Am J Roentgenol (AJR) 2008;191(1):145-150

14 Awai K, Inoue M, Yagyu Y et al. Moderate versus high concentration of contrast material for aortic and hepatic enhancement and tumor-to-liver contrast at multi-detector row CT. Radiology 2004;233:682-688

15 Herman S. Computed tomography contrast enhancement principles and the use of high-concentration contrast media. Comput Assist Tomogr 2004;28:S7-S11

16 Fenchel S, Fleiter TR, Aschoff AJ, et al. Effect of iodine concentration of contrast media on contrast enhancement in multislice CT of the pancreas. Br J Radiol 2004;77:821-830

17 Claussen CD, Banzer D, Pfretzschner C, et al. Bolus geometry and dynamics after intravenous contrast medium injection. Radiology 1984;153(2):365-368

18 Cademartiri F, van der Lugt A, Luccichenti G, et al. Parameters affecting bolus geometry in CT: A review. J Comput Assist Tomogr 2002;26(4):598-607

19 Ho LM, Nelson RC, DeLong DM. Determining contrast medium dose and rate on basis of lean body weight: Does this strategy improve patient-to-patient uniformity of hepatic enhancement during multi-detector row CT? Radiology 2007;243:431-437

20 Bae KT, Tran HQ, Heiken JP. Uniform vascular contrast enhancement and reduced contrast medium volume achieved by using exponentially decelerated contrast material injection method. Radiology 2004;231:732-736

21 Ichikawa T, Erturk SM, Araki T. Multiphasic contrast-enhanced multidetector-row CT of liver: contrast-enhancement theory and practical scan protocol with a combination of fixed injection duration and patients' body-weight-tailored dose of contrast material. Eur J Radiol 2006;58:165-176

22 Thomsen HS, Bush WH. Treatment of the adverse effects of contrast media. Acta Radiol 1998;39:212-218

23 Aspelin P, Aubry P, Fransson S-G, et al. Nephrotoxic effects in high-risk patients undergoing angiography. N Engl J Med 2003;348:491-499

24 Liss P, Persson PB, Hansell P, et al. Renal failure in 57 925 patients undergoing coronary procedures using iso-osmolar or low-osmolar contrast media. Kidney Int 2006;70(10):1811-1817

25 Persson PB, Hansell P, Liss P. Pathophysiology of contrast medium-induced nephropathy. Kidney Int 2005;68:14-22

26 Thomsen HS, Morcos SK. In which patients should serum creatinine be measured before iodinated contrast medium administration? Eur Radiol 2005;15:749-754

27 Thomsen HS, Morcos SK. Contrast media and the kidney: European Society of Urogenital Radiology (ESUR) guidelines. Br J Radiol 2003;76:513-518

28 Heller CA, Knapp J, Halliday J, et al. Failure to demonstrate contrast nephrotoxicity. Med J Aust 1991;155:329-332

29 Rao QA, Newhouse JH. Risk of nephropathy after intravenous administration of contrast material: a critical literature analysis. Radiology 2006;239:392-397

30 Katzberg RW and Barrett BJ. Risk of iodinated contrast material-induced nephropathy with intravenous administration. Radiology 2007;243:622-628

[31] Newhouse JH, Kho D, Rao QA, Starren J. Frequency of Serum Creatinine Changes in the Absence of Iodinated Contrast Material: Implications for Studies of Contrast Nephrotoxicity. AJR 2008;191:376-82

[32] Katzberg RW, Lamba R. Contrast-induced nephropathy after intravenous administration: fact or fiction? Radiol Clin North Am 2009;47:789-800

[33] Solomon RJ, Natarajan MK, Doucet S et al. Cardiac Angiography in Renally Impaired Patients (CARE) study: a randomized double-blind trial of contrast-induced nephropathy in patients with chronic kidney disease. Circulation 2007;115:3189-96

[34] Wessely R, Koppara T, Bradaric C et al. Choice of contrast medium in patients with impaired renal function undergoing percutaneous coronary intervention. Circ Cardiovasc Interv 2009;2:430-7

[35] Laskey W, Aspelin P, Davidson C et al. Nephrotoxicity of iodixanol versus iopamidol in patients with chronic kidney disease and diabetes mellitus undergoing coronary angiographic procedures. Am Heart J 2009;158:822-8

[36] Juergens CP, Winter JP, Nguyen-Do P et al. Nephrotoxic effects of iodixanol and iopromide in patients with abnormal renal function receiving N-acetylcysteine and hydration before coronary angiography and intervention: a randomized trial. Intern Med J 2009;39:25-31.

[37] Jost G, Pietsch H, Sommer J et al. Retention of iodine and expression of biomarkers for renal damage in the kidney after application of iodinated contrast media in rats. Invest Radiol 2009;44:114-23

[38] Seeliger E, Flemming B, Wronski T et al. Viscosity of contrast media perturbs renal hemodynamics. J Am Soc Nephrol 2007;18:2912-20

[39] Jost G, Pietsch H, Lengsfeld P, Hutter J, Sieber MA. The impact of the viscosity and osmolality of iodine contrast agents on renal elimination. Invest Radiol 2010;45:255-61

Cardiovascular and Body Radiology
DSCT Applications

Cardiac
Coronary CT Angiography

Dan Han
Bo He
Li Wu

Imaging Centre
Kunming Medical College
Kunming, Yunnan, China

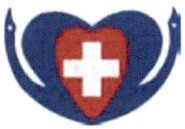

Cardiac
Coronary CT Angiography

Basic considerations

Excellent coronary artery imaging could be obtained with DSCT without heart rate control. It is important to choose the right amount and injection rate of contrast agent for a patient. In order to reduce radiation dose, several techniques can be employed. They include the ECG-based tube current modulation, careDose 4D or minDose activation, a reduction of tube voltage to 100 kV, attenuation-based tube current modulation; 100 kV/180 mAs may be considered in patients with low body mass index (BMI < 25) and step-and-shoot (SAS) mode.

Scan Parameters

Scan mode	Dual Source, ECG-gated
Heart rate control	not necessary
Scan area	mid pulmonary artery to below heart
Scan direction	cranio-caudal
Scan time	~5–12 s, depending on heart rate*
Tube voltage	120 kV
Tube current	380 mAs/rotation *
Dose modulation	ECG-pulsing (details in Table on page 22)
$CTDI_{vol}$	~50–60 mGy, depending on heart rate*
Rotation time	0.33 s
Pitch	0.2–0.5, depending on heart rate
Slice collimation	0.6 mm
Acquisition	64 x 0.6 mm
Slice width	0.75 mm
Reconstruction increment	0.4 mm
Reconstruction kernel	B26f*

* Asian Adaptation by Kunming Medical College
Higher image quality leads to slightly increased values for mAs/rot. and $CTDI_{vol}$.

Tricks

Images are most frequently reconstructed in 0.75 mm slice thickness and slice increment of 0.4–0.5 mm and the dedicated kernel B26f, which is used to perform three-dimensional (3D), MIPs and curved MPRs and to evaluate coronary arteries. For heart rates lower than 90 bpm automatic best phase selection can usually satisfy clinical demands.

Pitfalls

When the tube voltage is reduced to 100 kV, CT values in the coronary arteries segment will be higher than with 120 kV. In patients with high body mass index (BMI > 30), it may be useful to increase contrast flow rate and to employ the CardioObese mode.

Contrast Injection Protocol

	Iodine concentration 370 mg I/ml
Injection scheme	Monophasic
Iodine delivery rate	1.85 g/s
CM volume	5 ml/s for duration of scan, ≥ 50 ml
CM flow rate	5 ml/s
Body weight adaptation	no
Bolus timing	test bolus **
Bolus tracking threshold	n.a.
ROI position	ascending aorta
Scan delay	peak time plus 2 s
Saline flush volume	60 ml
Saline injection rate	5 ml/s
Needle size	18 G
Injection site	antecubital vein

** Depending on the preference of the individual site, bolus tracking can be used as an alternative

Case 1
Excluding Coronary Artery Heart Disease in Dyspnea (Normal Coronary Arteries)

Case history

A 50-year-old male presented with 1 year of dyspnea, 1 month of palpitation, and 3 days of exacerbation. The dynamic ECG was suspected positive. ECG and ECHO were both negative.

The purpose is to exclude coronary artery heart disease.

Diagnosis / Differential diagnosis

Suspected positive of DECG suggested that myocardial ischemia caused by coronary artery stenosis or spasm might exist. The diagnosis of cardiomyopathy or coronary artery heart disease should be considered. The differential diagnosis depended on coronary arteriography. CTA displayed normal coronary artery.

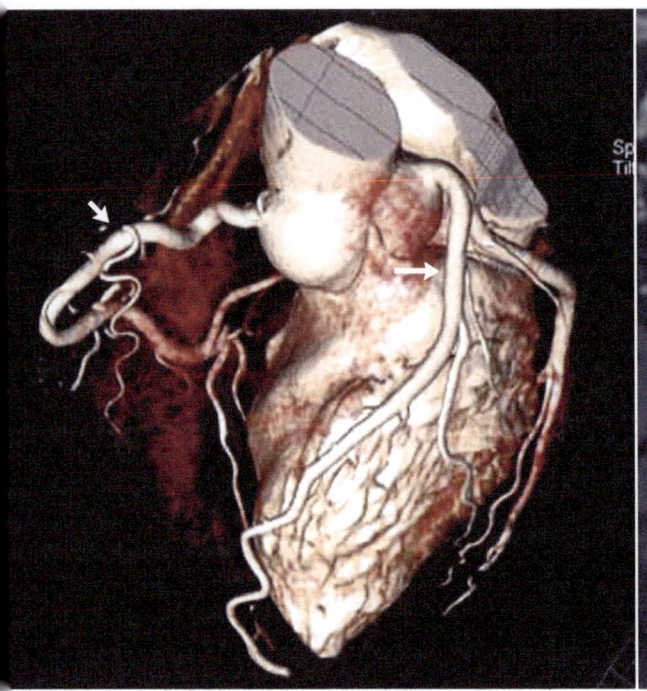

[1] VRT of the heart and coronary arteries, here showing normal LAD (large arrow) and RCA (small arrow).

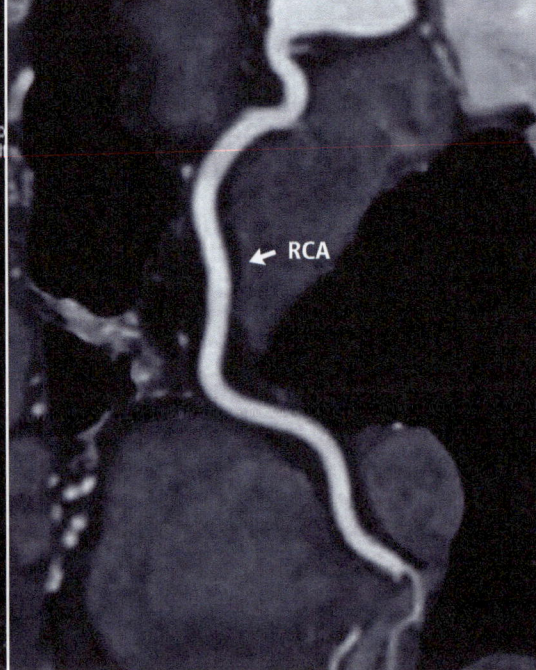

[2–4] RCA, LAD, LCX
CPR images of the coronary arteries demonstrate that arteries are regular and smooth without stenosis and plaques.

Findings

This patient's heart rate was 68 bpm. Both VRT and CPR images demonstrated that the coronary arteries were free from stenosis and atherosclerosis. No invasive angiography was necessary.

Take-home message

High-quality images clearly demonstrate coronary artery without any moving artifact. Coronary artery diseases are excluded and the invasive coronary arteriography is not necessary.

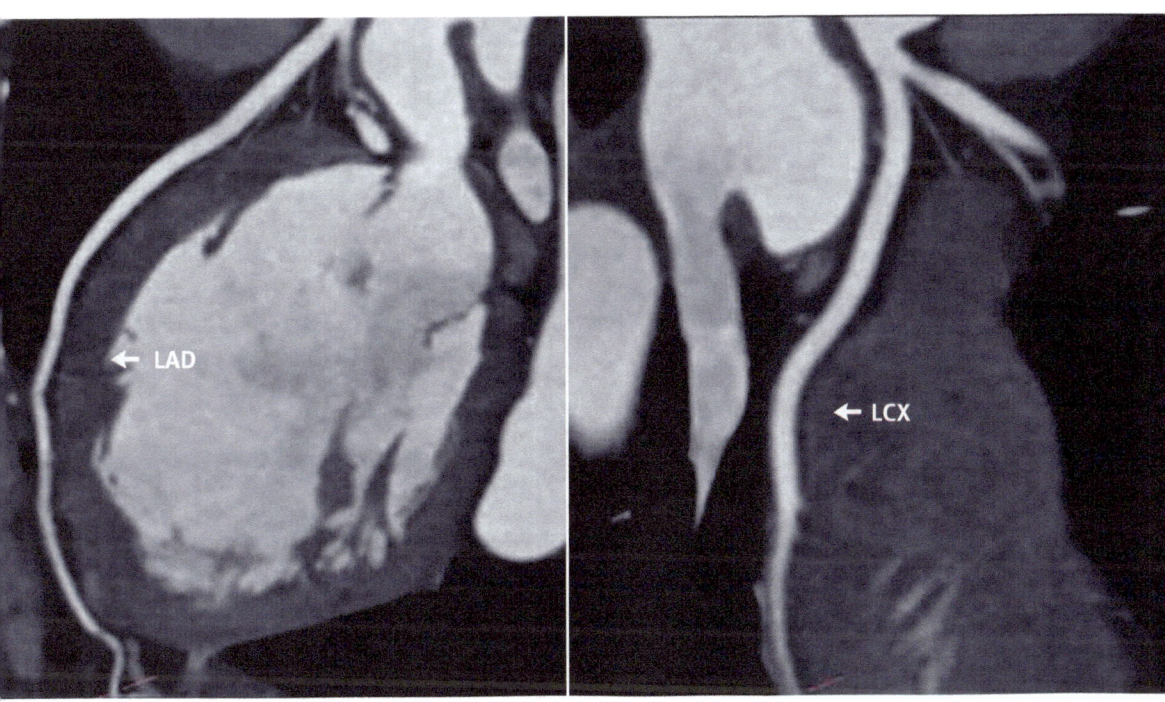

Case 2
A Total Occlusion in the LCX

Case history

A 66-year-old male presented with atypical chest pain and chest tightness for 1 month.

Diagnosis / Differential diagnosis

A relatively long, chronic total occlusion of the middle CX coronary artery was found.

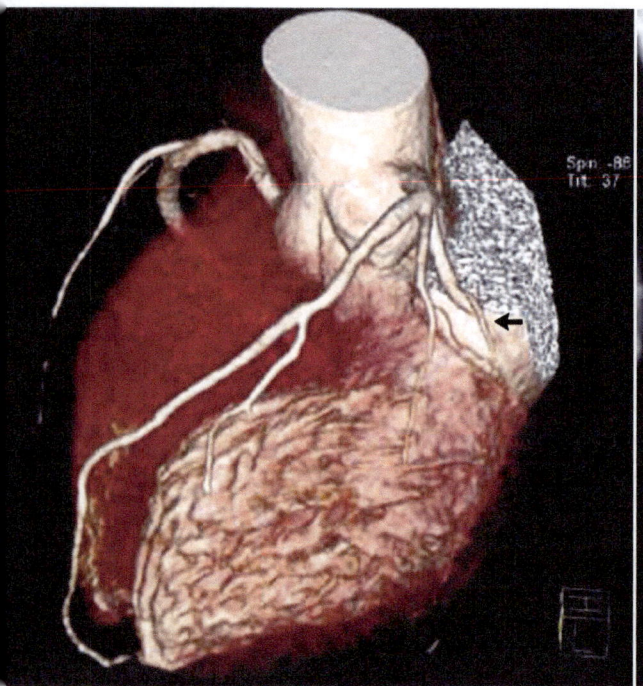

[1] VRT: Severe stenosis at middle segment of CX.

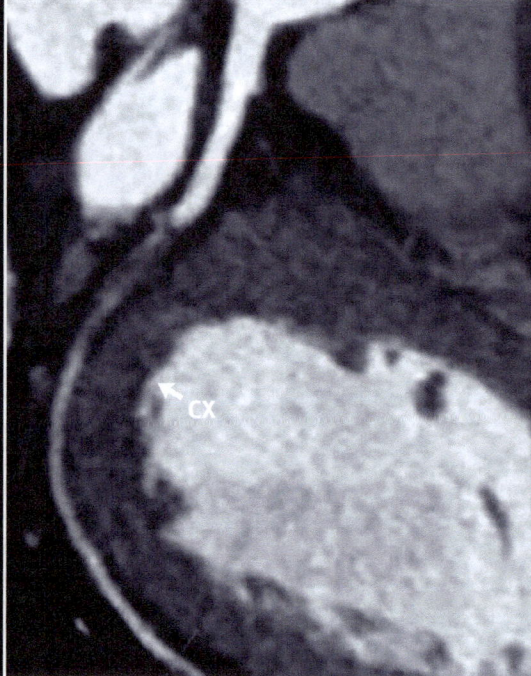

[2–3] CPR: The component of plaque and stenosed degree shown on CT are in accordance with those on IVUS (arrow).

Findings

There was a soft plaque at the middle segment of CX and the lumen was occluded; VRT, MIP and CPR demonstrated occlusion and interruption of this vessel which had no calcification. The remaining coronary arteries were normal. DSA also confirmed the interruption of the middle CX, the plaque shape, component and stenosed location shown on IVUS were in accordance with those on CT. PCI was performed successfully.

Take-home message

CT signs are in accordance with the findings on IVUS and DSA. CTA also gives the indication that the cause of stenosis is extremely low density soft plaque which makes it easier to insert a catheter through the lumen and hence improve the possibility of successful intervention. Coronary CTA plays a role as important as "eyes" in interventional operation.

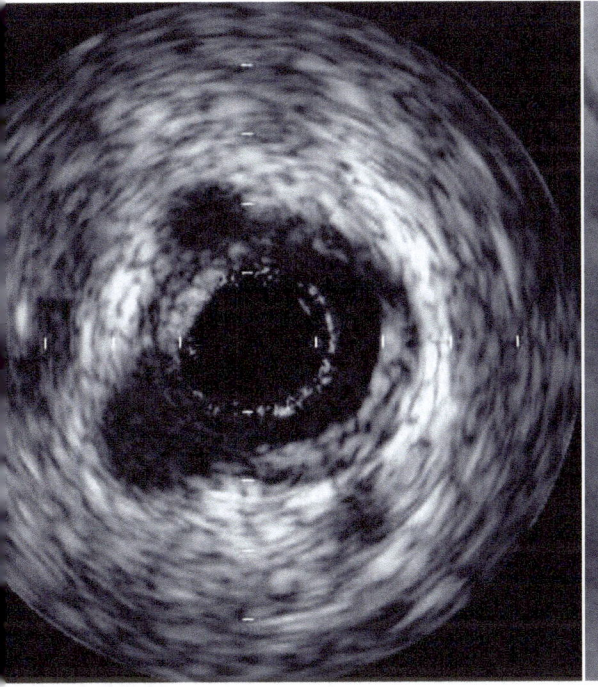 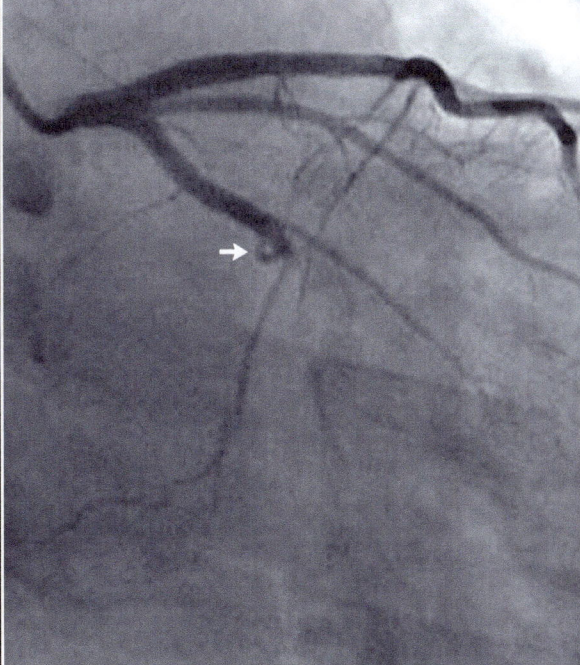

[4] DSA: Complete interruption at proximal CX (arrow).

Cardiac
Coronary Stents

Liu Ming
Feng Yun
Xue Jianping
Li Yuhua

Department of Radiology
Xinhua Hospital
Shanghai, China

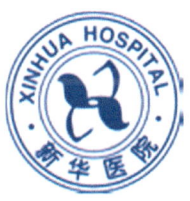

Cardiac
Coronary Stents

Basic considerations

You can use an image protocol with maximal spatial and temporal resolution for optimized image quality, similar to the protocol used for standard coronary CT angiography. You can also use an injection protocol similar to the protocol used for standard coronary CT angiography. Reconstruction with a sharp kernel (B46) may help to better visualize stent lumen. Image reconstructions should include curved and multiplanar reformations. [1]

Scan Parameters

Scan mode	Dual Source, ECG-gated
Heart rate control	not necessary
Scan area	mid pulmonary artery to below heart
Scan direction	cranio-caudal
Scan time	~5–12 s, depending on heart rate *
Tube voltage	120 kV
Tube current	380 mAs/rotation *
Dose modulation	ECG-pulsing (details in Table on page 22)
CTDI$_{vol}$	~50–60 mGy, depending on heart rate *
Rotation time	0.33 s
Pitch	0.2–0.5, depending on heart rate
Slice collimation	0.6 mm
Acquisition	64 x 0.6 mm
Slice width	0.75 mm *
Reconstruction increment	0.5 mm *
Reconstruction kernel	B46f

* Asian Adaptation by Shanghai Xinhua Hospital
Higher image quality leads to slightly increased values for mAs/rot. and CTDI$_{vol}$.

Tricks

To evaluate stented coronary artery segments, we recommend a kernel with stronger edge-enhancing characteristics (sharp B46 kernel versus soft B26 kernel). This usually increases the visible stent lumen and may help to avoid false positive readings of stent obstruction. [1]

Pitfalls

Due to beam-hardening effects, which cause increased CT values adjacent to the stent, stents appear significantly larger in CT images than their actual size. A decrease in density is generally observed from the periphery towards the center of the stent lumen. Therefore, the size of the vessel lumen appears artificially reduced in a stented coronary artery segment. [1]

Contrast Injection Protocol

	Iodine concentration 370 mg I/ml
Injection scheme	Monophasic
Iodine delivery rate	1.85 g/s
CM volume	5 ml/s for duration of scan, ≥ 50 ml
CM flow rate	5 ml/s
Body weight adaptation	no
Bolus timing	test bolus **
Bolus tracking threshold	n.a.
ROI position	left ventricle
Scan delay	peak time
Saline flush volume	50 ml
Saline injection rate	5 ml/s
Needle size	18 G
Injection site	antecubital vein

** Depending on the preference of the individual site, bolus tracking can be used as an alternative

[1] S. Ruehm, C. Arellano, C. Panknin in [1]

Case 1
Stent in CX

Case history

52-year-old male with CAD underwent PCI two years ago and showed ischemic symptoms post stent placement in CX.

Diagnosis / Differential diagnosis

The stent in the proximal CX was widely patent. The lumen of the proximal LAD showed signs of stenosis. There was a small plaque in the proximal aspect of the diagonal branch.

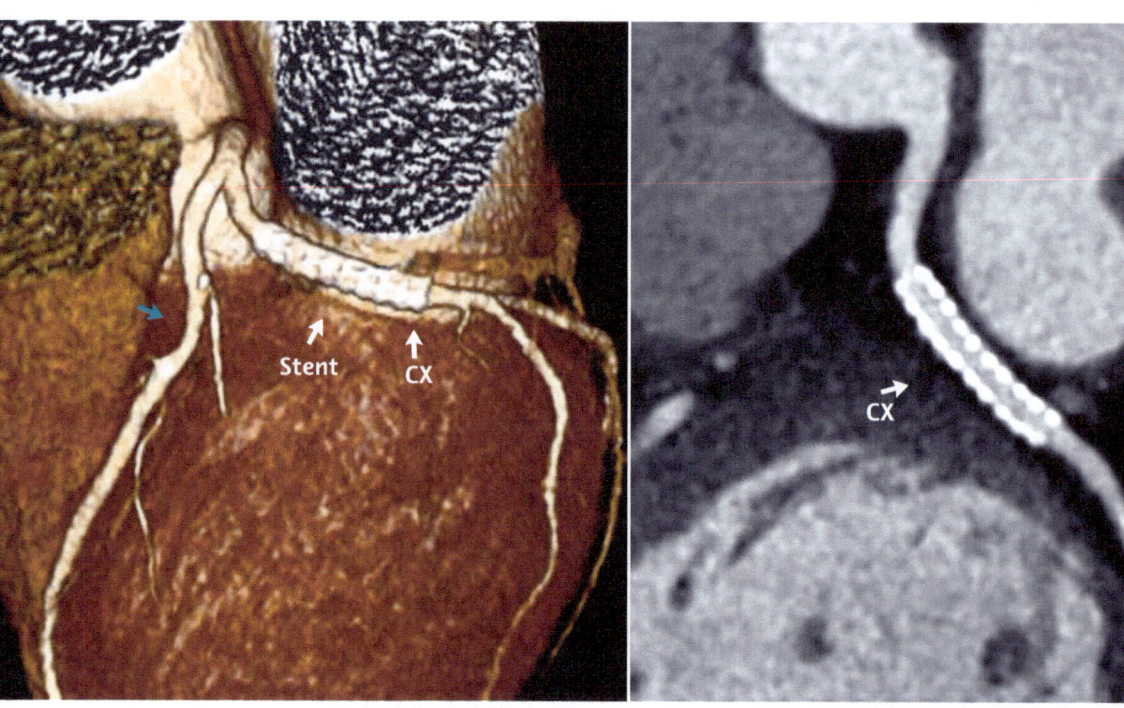

[1] Volume-rendered 3D reconstruction shows stent in proximal CX and also shows the luminal stenosis in LAD (blue arrow).

[2] Curved reformatted image of CX (reconstruction with sharp B46 kernel) shows a widely patent stent.

Findings

The lumen of the stent in the CX showed homogeneous opacification consistent with stent patency. A non-calcified plaque was seen in the proximal LAD and the lumen showed mild stenosis. A small calcified plaque was noted immediately proximal to the diagonal branch without significant luminal stenosis.

Take-home message

The post-processing techniques such as curved reformations combined with a sharp reconstruction (B46 kernel) are available for the evaluation of the in-stent lumen. Homogeneous opacification of the lumen suggests a widely patent stent. CT angiogram can easily reveal the peripheral plaque of coronary arteries based on the high spatial resolution.

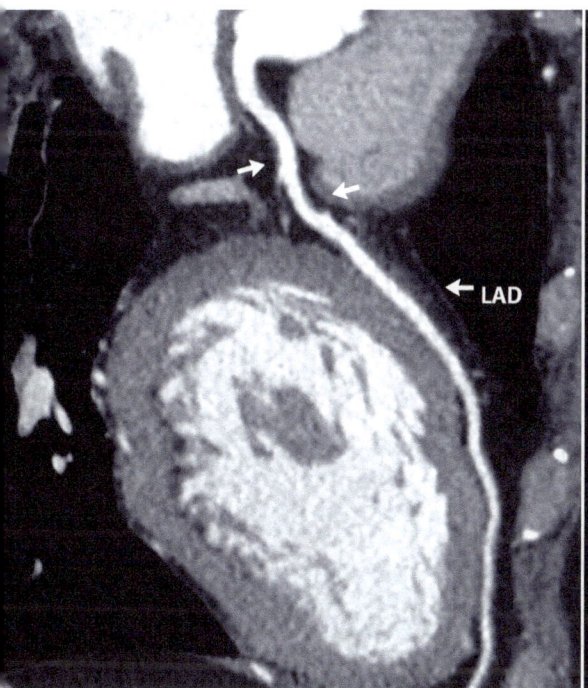

[3] Curved reformatted image of LAD shows signs of stenosis. Note non-calcified plaque proximal to LAD and the mild luminal stenosis.

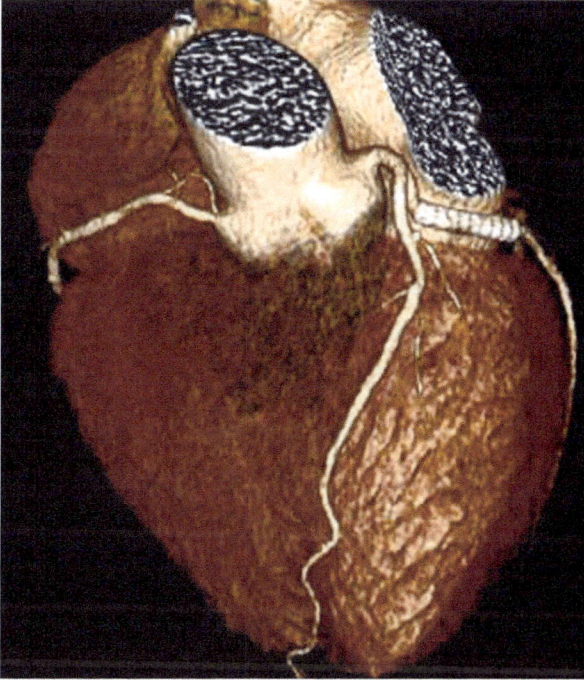

[4] Volume-rendered 3D reconstruction display of coronary angiogram (RCA, LAD, CX with stent).

Case 2
Stents in LAD and RCA

Case history

A 45-year-old male showed angina-like symptoms. He had a history of percutaneous coronary intervention (PCI) and stent placement in the left anterior descending coronary artery (LAD) and right coronary artery (RCA). The patient was scheduled for a follow-up study to assess stent patency and overall situation of coronary arteries.

Diagnosis / Differential diagnosis

The DSCT coronary angiogram demonstrated no evidence of in-stent restenosis in the stents of proximal LAD and distal RCA. A myocardial bridge was detected in the mid-to-distal segment of LAD.

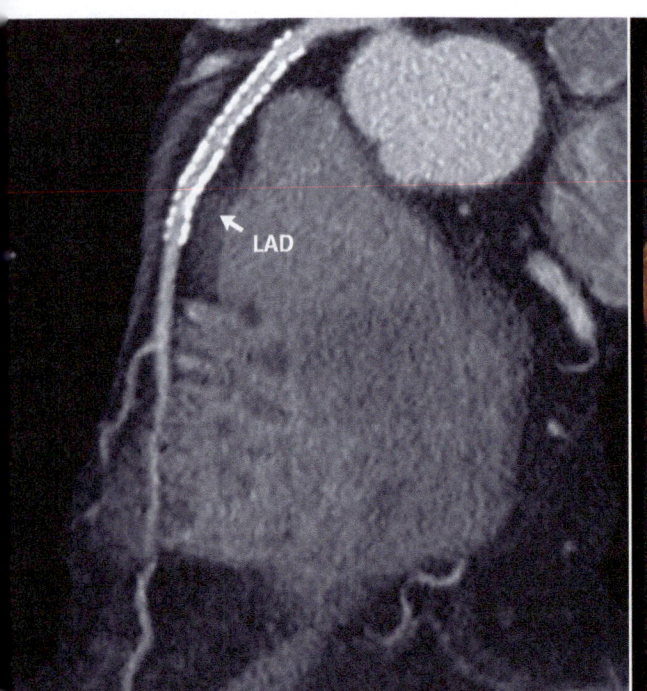

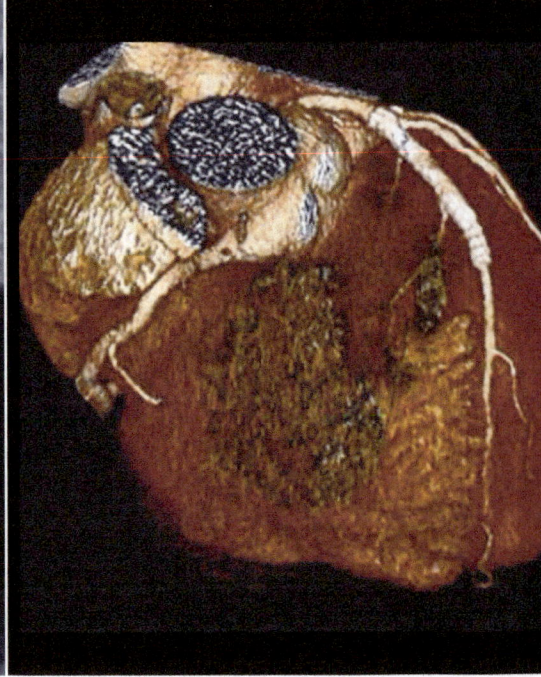

[1] Maximum intensity projection (MIP) image shows stent (arrow) in proximal segment of left anterior descending coronary artery (LAD).

[2] Three-dimensional volume-rendered (VRT) image demonstrates the stent in proximal LAD.

Findings

The DSCT coronary angiogram allowed reliable visualization of the coronary lumen inside the stent, thereby reliably excluding the presence of in-stent restenosis. This scan clearly demonstrated the absence of in-stent restenosis and neointimal hyperplasia. No significantly obstructive stenoses were shown on the DSCT scan. The patient had a heart rate of 78 bpm during the scan. The image quality was still good, there were no artifacts and beam-hardening artifacts.

Take-home message

Dual Source CT coronary angiogram has the ability to be widely used for ruling out the presence of in-stent narrowing or occlusion in follow-up patients after PCI, even without the need for pre-scan beta-blockers.

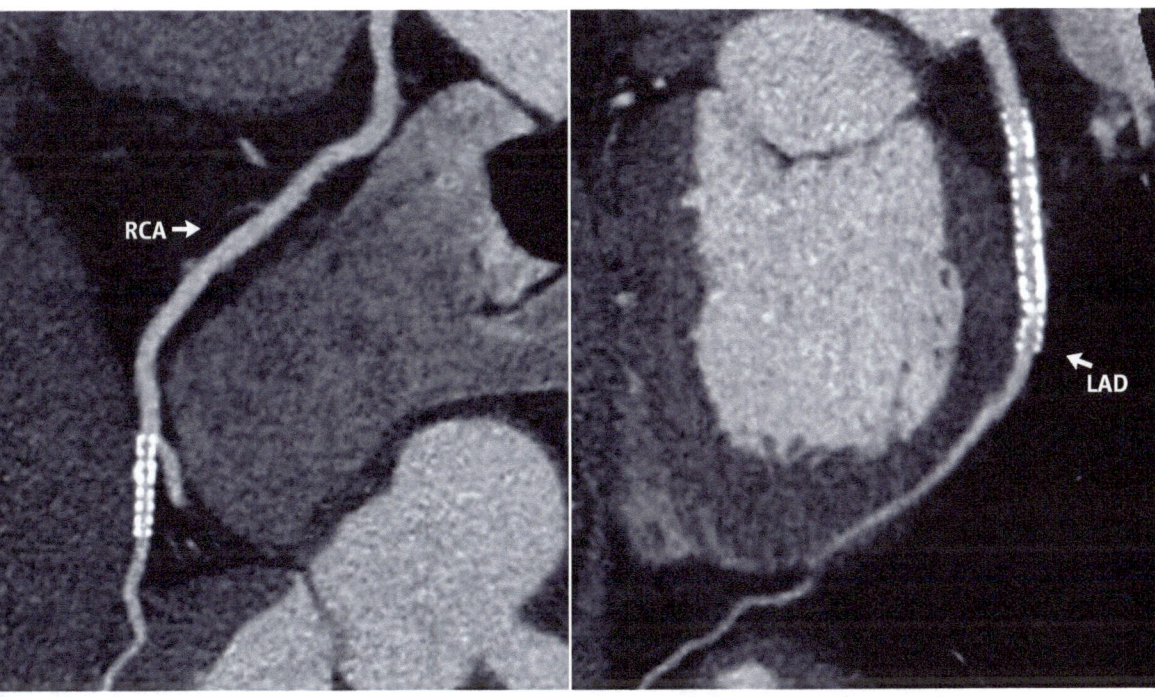

[3] Curved multiplanar reconstruction (MPR) of the right coronary artery (RCA) (arrow) with no significant in-stent restenosis.

[4] Curved MPR image of the LAD shows stent patency due to homogeneous contrast enhancement inside the lumen of this long stent (arrow).

Cardiac
Coronary CTA
in Obese Patients

Song Lan
Wang Yining
Zhang Zhuhua
Kong Lingyan
Jin Zhengyu

Department of Radiology
Peking Union Medical College Hospital
Beijing, China

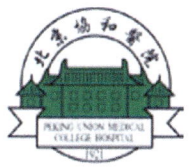

Cardiac
Coronary CTA in Obese Patients

Basic considerations

Consider using CardioObese™ mode for BMI ≥ 35 kg/m^2. Obese patients have increased noise due to photon scattering. CardioObese™ mode improves signal-to-noise. Temporal resolution is decreased to 165 ms/slice but the signal strength is improved. Beta-blockers are therefore administered to ensure a heart rate during acquisition of less than 65 bpm.

Contrast flow rate can also be increased to improve contrast-to-noise ratio. [1]

Scan Parameters

Scan mode	Dual Source obese mode, ECG-gated *
Heart rate control	< 70 bpm preferable
Scan area	mid pulmonary artery to below heart
Scan direction	cranio-caudal
Scan time	~8–10 s, depending on heart rate *
Tube voltage	120 kV
Tube current	420 mAs/rotation
Dose modulation	ECG-pulsing on *
CTDI$_{vol}$	~65 mGy, depending on heart rate *
Rotation time	0.33 s
Pitch	0.2–0.5, depending on heart rate
Slice collimation	0.6 mm
Acquisition	64 x 0.6 mm
Slice width	0.75 mm
Reconstruction increment	0.4 mm
Reconstruction kernel	B26f, B46f in case of excessive calcification

* Asian Adaptation by PUMC, Beijing
In case of obese patients, the system default parameters for the ECG-pulsing window are used instead of user-defined fixed ECG-pulsing widths. This results in slightly decreased dose values.

Tricks

If the heart rate is ≤ 65 bpm, the 165 ms reconstruction is generally best. Higher iodine concentration should be used if a flow rate of 6 ml/s cannot be achieved. [1]

Pitfalls

Inadequate heart rate control. Poor sensing of ECG signal due to body mass. Difficulty with IV site due to subcutaneous fat. BMI > 50 kg/m^2 has not been consistently tested. Scan should probably not be performed in this population if heart rate is > 80 bpm. [1]

Contrast Injection Protocol

	Iodine concentration 370 mg I/ml
Injection scheme	Monophasic
Iodine delivery rate	1.8 g/s
CM volume	75 ml (add 10 ml for 5 BMI points)
CM flow rate	4.9 ml/s
Body weight adaptation	yes
Bolus timing	bolus tracking **
Bolus tracking threshold	120 HU
ROI position	ascending aorta
Scan delay	10 s
Saline flush volume	60 ml
Saline injection rate	4.9 ml/s
Needle size	18 G
Injection site	antecubital vein

** Depending on the preference of the individual site, test bolus can be used as an alternative

[1] K. Chinnaiyan, R. Gentry, G. Raff in [1]

Case 1
DSCT in an Obese Man: Chest Pain and Dyspnea

Case history

A 50-year-old obese male (BMI of 37 kg/m^2) presented with dyspnea on excercise and atypical chest discomfort. He was under the treatment of insulin injection for type 2 diabetes mellitus.

Diagnosis/Differential diagnosis

Mild stenosis of middle LAD with eccentric calcified plaque was detected. Cardiac structure and function were normal. There was no CT evidence of valvular abnormalities. Non-cardiac structures were unremarkable.

Findings

The average heart rate during acquisition was 52 bpm (50–56 bpm). The image quality of the scan was excellent. All coronary segments were visualized well. Compared to temporal resolution of 83 ms, images reconstructed at a temporal resolution of 165 ms were superior in quality, with

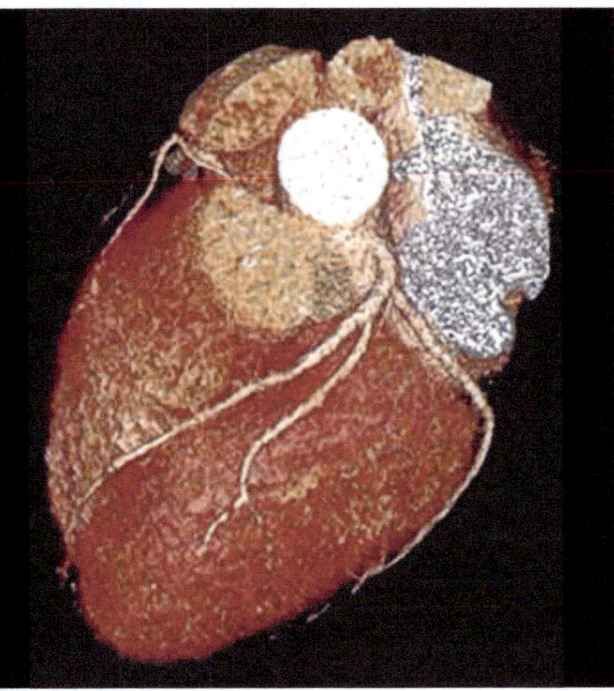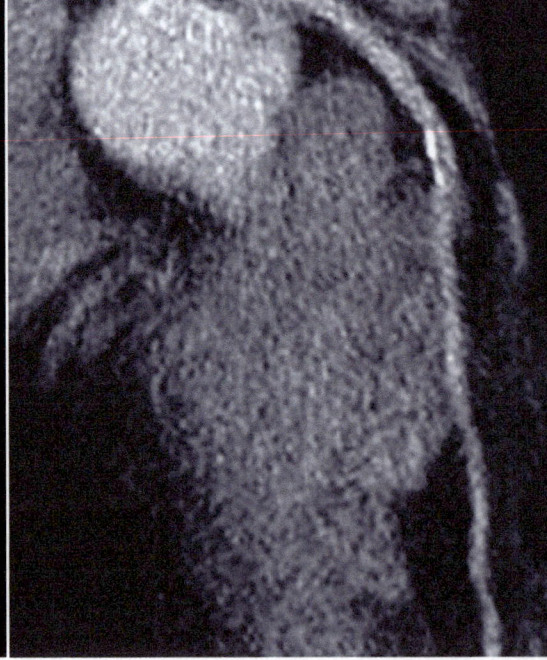

[1–2] Reconstruction at temporal resolution of 83 ms (Noise = 29[SD], contrast-to-noise ratio (CNR) = 8.3, signal-to-noise ratio (SNR) = 9.9).

higher signal-to-noise ratio (SNR) and contrast-to-noise ratio (CNR).

Take-home message

Use of the Cardio-Obese protocol of DSCT and proper management of contrast administration allows excellent visualization of coronary arteries in the majority of this population (BMI > 35 kg/m^2). Heart rate control (70 bpm) is essential in this subset of patients. Reconstruction at a lower temporal resolution (165 ms) results in better image quality when heart rate during acquisition is below 65 bpm. Administering the higher contrast bolus at a higher infusion rate can result in higher CNR, further enhancing the image quality of the scan. For further improvement in image quality, reconstruction at various temporal resolutions (83 ms to 165 ms) and proper adjustment of the contrast injection protocol is recommended.

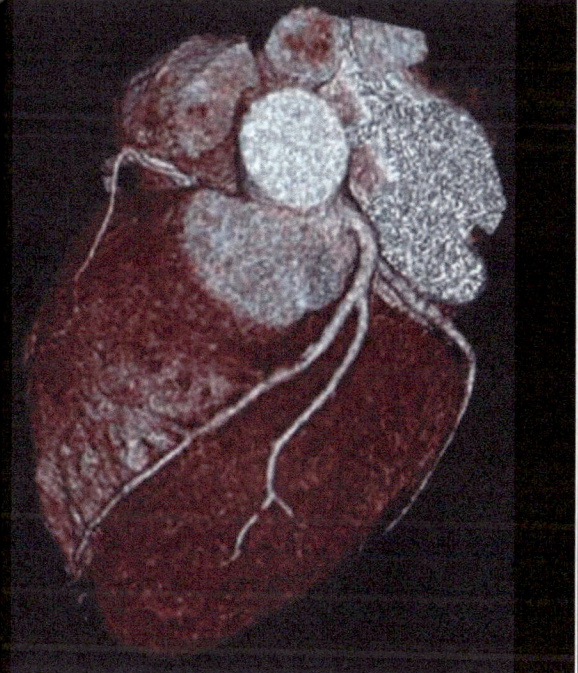
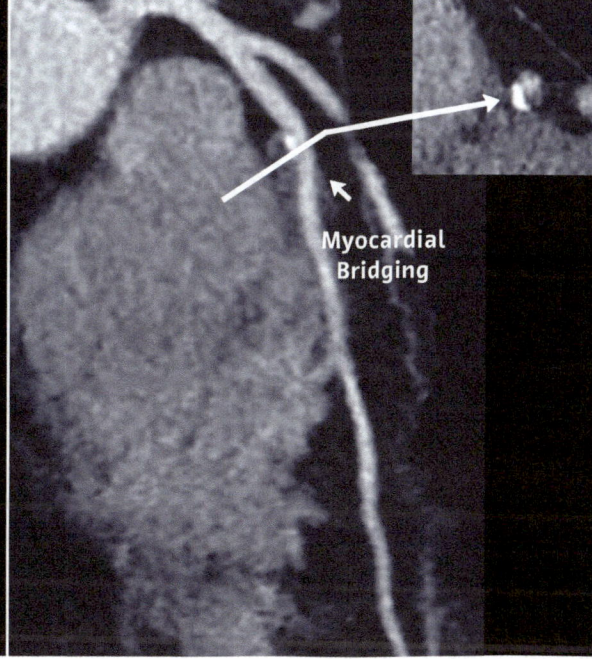

Myocardial
Bridging

[3–4] Reconstruction at temporal resolution of 165 ms
(Noise = 19[SD], CNR = 12.8, SNR = 15.4).

Case 2
DSCT in an Obese Man: Chest Pain

Case history

A 29-year-old obese male presented with a BMI of 39.2 kg/m², his body weight was 120 kg, at a height of 1.75 m. He presented with chest pain for more than 9 months and was clinically suspected of nodular polyarteritis. He was a smoker, about 10 cigarettes per day. He had hypertension, with the highest blood pressure of 180/120 mm Hg, under treatment with Metoprolol and Benazepril.

Diagnosis / Differential diagnosis

There was mild calcification (calcium score=33.3), and an irregular dilatation of multiple segments of coronary arteries, with low density substances attached to the LAD and right coronary wall, which was plaque or thrombus. The distal segment of the right coronary artery was obliterated. Three myocardial bridges were located at the middle and distal segment of LAD, two of them showed 60~70% stenosis of the coronary artery under the myocardial bridge. Cardiac size and function were normal.

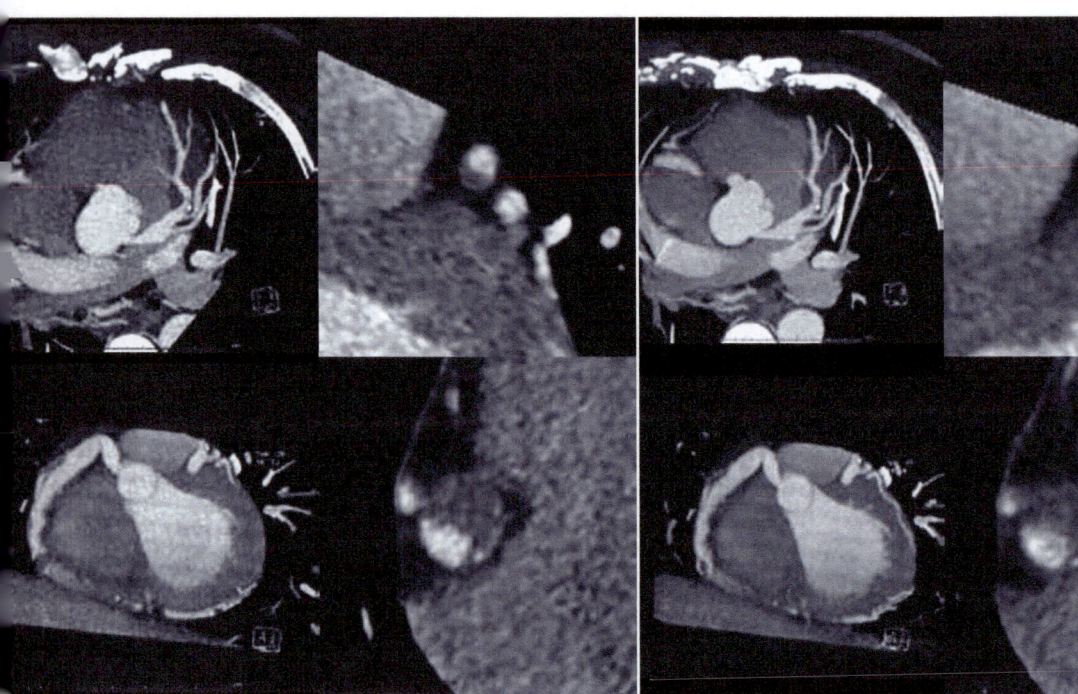

[1] Reconstruction at the temporal resolution of 83 ms.

[2] Reconstruction at the temporal resolution of 165 ms.

Findings

Heart rate during acquisition was 61 bpm (Range, 58–66 bpm). The image quality was good. Reconstruction at a lower temporal resolution (165 ms) provided a smoother image, for the reconstruction at a higher temporal resolution (83 ms), the margin of the cross-sectional image of the coronary artery was clearer, and the border between the lumen and the vessel wall was sharper.

Take-home message

Use of the Cardio-Obese protocol of DSCT and proper management of contrast administration allows excellent visualization of coronary arteries in obese patient. If the heart rate is < 70 bpm, both reconstructions at a lower temporal resolution (165 ms) and a higher temporal resolution provide good image quality of diagnostic value.

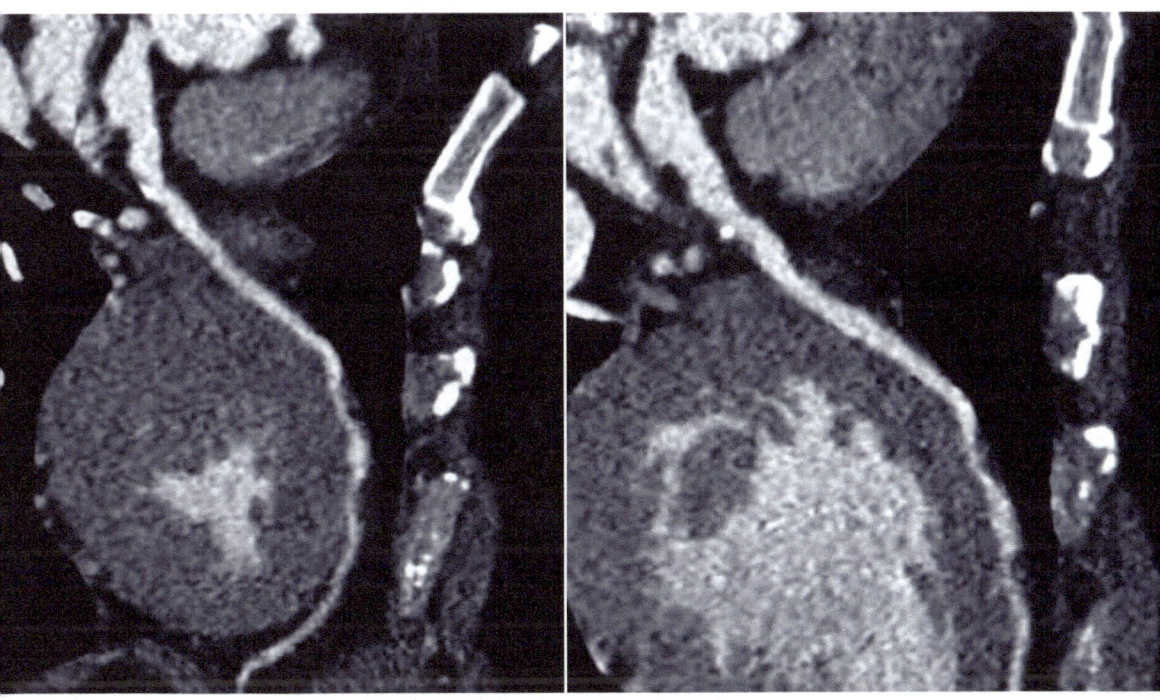

[3] Reconstruction at the temporal resolution of 83 ms (systolic phase).

[4] Reconstruction at the temporal resolution of 83 ms (diagnostic phase).

Cardiac
Valvular Function

Joon-Won Kang
Joon Beom Seo
Kyung-Hyun Do
Tae-Hwan Lim

Department of Radiology and Research Institute of
Radiology
Asan Medical Center
Seoul, Korea

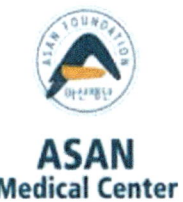

ASAN
Medical Center

Cardiac
Valvular Function

Basic considerations

The implementation of ECG-pulsing depends on the valvular disease of interest and should always take into account considerations about the increased radiation dose when not using ECG-pulsing. ECG-pulsing must be turned off when evaluating aortic stenosis or mitral regurgitation as it requires imaging in systole. ECG-pulsing should be switched on when analyzing aortic regurgitation, mitral stenosis or morphological abnormalities in patients with infective valvular endocarditis. Consider 100 kV / 330 mAs in patients with low body mass index, depending on the patient's habitus. In patients with high body mass index, it may be useful to increase contrast flow and to employ the CardioObese™ mode. [1]

Scan Parameters

Scan mode	Dual Source, ECG-gated
Heart rate control	not necessary
Scan area	whole chest *
Scan direction	cranio-caudal
Scan time	~14 s, depending on heart rate *
Tube voltage	100 kV *
Tube current	400 mAs/rotation *
Dose modulation	CARE Dose4D, no ECG-pulsing *
$CTDI_{vol}$	~45 mGy, depending on heart rate *
Rotation time	0.33 s
Pitch	0.2 – 0.5, depending on heart rate
Slice collimation	0.6 mm
Acquisition	64 x 0.6 mm
Slice width	0.75 mm
Reconstruction increment	0.4 mm
Reconstruction kernel	B26f / B30f *

* **Asian Adaptation by Asan Medical Center**
Due to the slimmer population in Asia, typically lower kV values at an adjusted quality ref. mAs/rot. level in combination with CARE Dose4D are used which leads to lower $CTDI_{vol}$ values.

Tricks

The scan range must be fitted to the respective indication: e.g. evaluation of the aortic valve should cover the aortic root to allow for geometric assessment of its dimensions. Patients should hold their breath in mild-inspiration. This should be trained on the scanner table immediately prior to the examination. [1]

Pitfalls

Images in several cardiac phases must be evaluated to define the phase with maximum opening or closing of the valve. Accurate multi-planar reformations exactly parallel and perpendicular to the respective valve must be performed. Valve opening areas and regurgitation orifice areas can be measured three times and averaged to yield more robust results. [1]

Contrast Injection Protocol

	Iodine concentration 370 mg I/ml
Injection scheme	Monophasic
Iodine delivery rate	1.85 g/s
CM volume	5 ml/s for duration of scan, ≥ 50 ml
CM flow rate	5 ml/s
Body weight adaptation	no
Bolus timing	bolus tracking **
Bolus tracking threshold	140 HU
ROI position	ascending aorta
Scan delay	2 s
Saline flush volume	60 ml
Saline injection rate	5 ml/s
Needle size	18 G
Injection site	antecubital vein

** Depending on the preference of the individual site, test bolus can be used as an alternative

[1] H. Alkahdi, S. Leschka, H. Scheffel, P. Stolzmann in [1]

Case 1
Prolapse of Anterior Leaflet of Bicuspid Aortic Valve

Case history

A 50-year-old male presented with fever and myalgia for 3 months. He had a history of spondylodiscitis of the lumbar spine. On the transthoracic echocardiography, aortic regurgitation and a bicuspid aortic valve with vegetation were found. His heart rate during the CT scan was 75 to 80 bpm.

Diagnosis / Differential diagnosis

Bicuspid aortic valve showed aortic insufficiency. An infective endocarditis was detected. A cyst at the mitral valve anterior leaflet was found.

Findings

There was an aortic valve with an anterior-posterior type of fusion of right and left leaflets. An out-pouching lesion at the left side commissure of the aortic valve was regarded as abscess. In

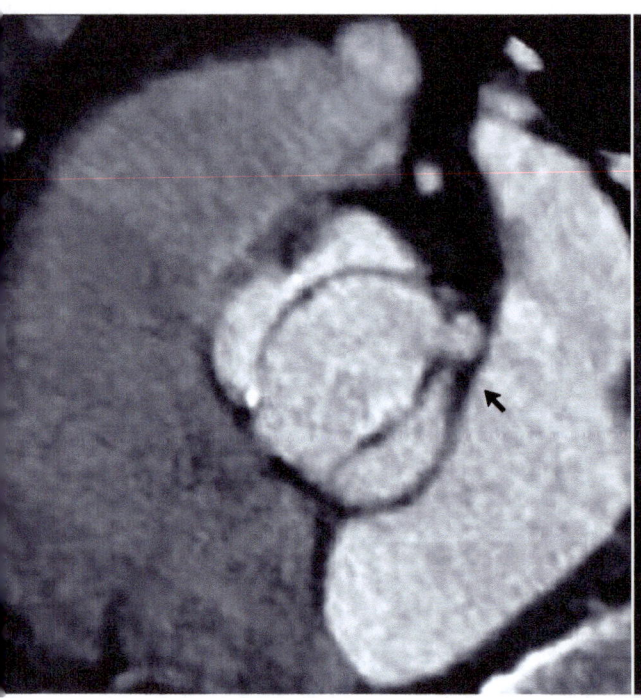 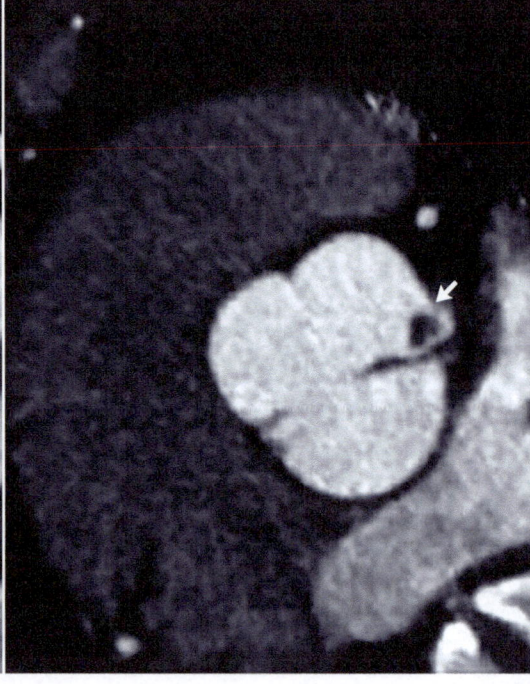

[1] En face view of the aortic valve at 70% of R-R interval shows bicuspid aortic valve with out-pouching lesion at the left commissure of the valve (arrow).

[2] En face view of the aortic valve at 10% of R-R interval shows coaptation failure of the bicuspid aortic valve. Small nodular lesion is seen on the inferior part of the anterior leaflet (arrow).

addition, there was a small nodular lesion at the inferior margin of the anterior leaflet which was regarded as the vegetation. There was coaptation failure of the aortic valve caused by prolapse of the anterior leaflet. An ovoid-shaped, thin-walled lesion was detected at the atrial aspect of anterior leaflet of the mitral valve. It did not move into the left ventricle, and there was no mitral valve insufficiency.

Take-home message

With optimal injection protocol and scan protocol, the morphology and motion of the bicuspid aortic valve can be assessed very well. Tumor lesion of the mitral valve as well as morphology and motion can be assessed effectively with DSCT and an appropriate contrast media injection protocol.

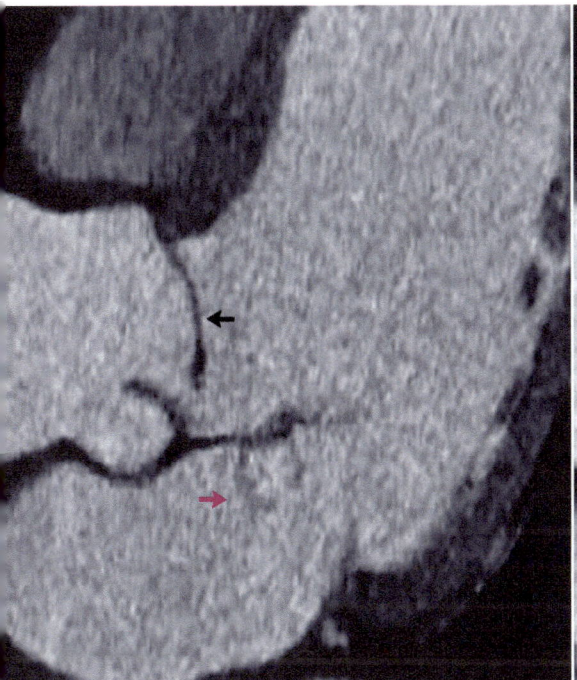

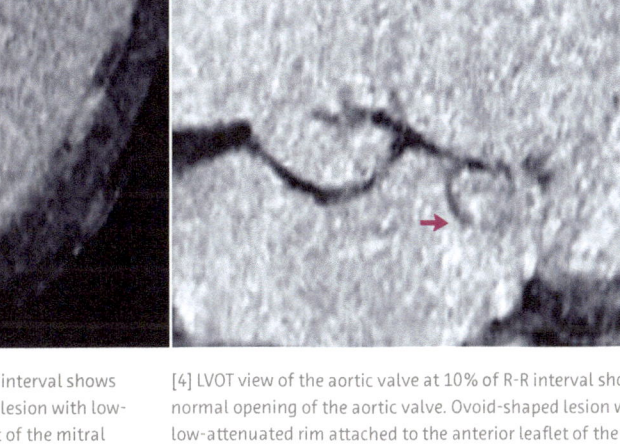

[3] LVOT view of the aortic valve at 70% of R-R interval shows prolapse of the anterior leaflet. Ovoid-shaped lesion with low-attenuated rim attached to the anterior leaflet of the mitral valve is seen (pink arrow).

[4] LVOT view of the aortic valve at 10% of R-R interval shows normal opening of the aortic valve. Ovoid-shaped lesion with low-attenuated rim attached to the anterior leaflet of the mitral valve is seen (pink arrow).

Case 2
Rheumatic Aortic Valve Steno-insufficiency and Mitral Valve Stenosis

Case history

A 40-year-old female presented with systolic ejection murmur for 3 years. Trans-aortic valve peak velocity increased from 4.5 m/s to 5.1 m/s, and the pressure gradient was increased from 80 (maximum)/46 (mean) mm Hg to 105/61 mm Hg on the echocardiography follow-up from 2005 to 2008. She had a history of percutaneous mitral valvuloplasty 10 years ago. Her heart rate during the CT scan was 46 to 55 bpm (mean 48 bpm).

Diagnosis / Differential diagnosis

An aortic valve steno-insufficiency probably of rheumatic origin was found. In addition, doming of the mitral valve with limited motion of the posterior leaflet was detected.

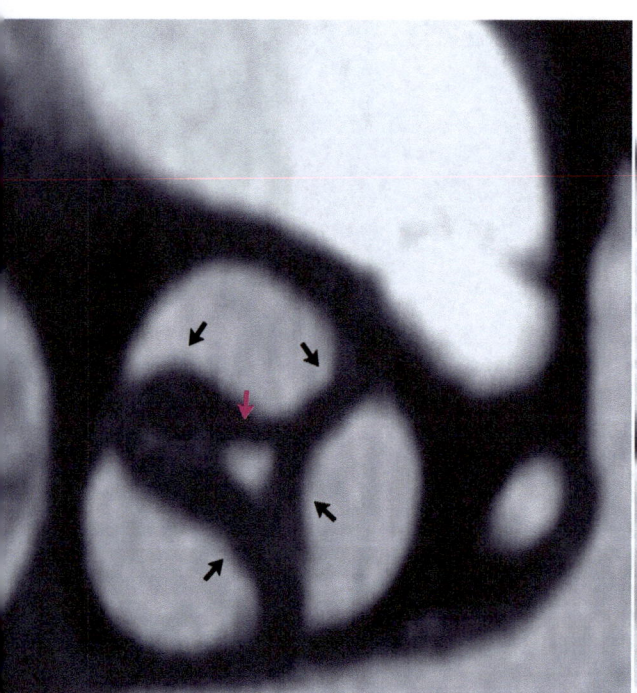 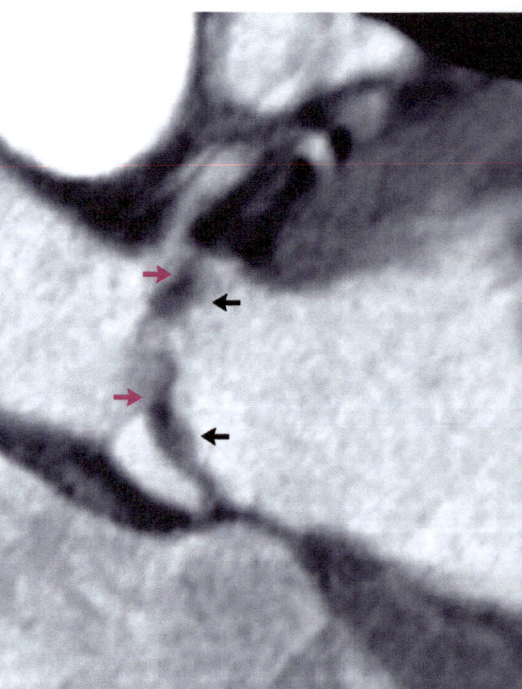

[1] LVOT view at the 70% R-R interval shows diffuse thickening of the aortic valve (dark arrows). Central coaptation of the aortic valve is seen (pink arrow).

[2] LVOT view at the 10% R-R interval shows diffuse thickening of the aortic valve (dark arrows). Doming of the aortic valve is seen (pink arrows).

Findings

On the mid-diastolic phase, en face view of the aortic valve image, aortic valve was thickened and not completely closed. On the systolic phase image, the aortic valve showed doming and had opening limitation. On the mid-diastolic phase 4-chamber view image, the anterior leaflet of the mitral valve showed doming, and the posterior leaflet was not completely open. Both leaflets of the mitral valve were thickened.

Take-home message

With optimum injection protocol and scan protocol, the morphology and motion of the aortic valve can be assessed very well. Mitral valve morphology and motion can be assessed effectively with DSCT and the appropriate contrast media injection protocol.

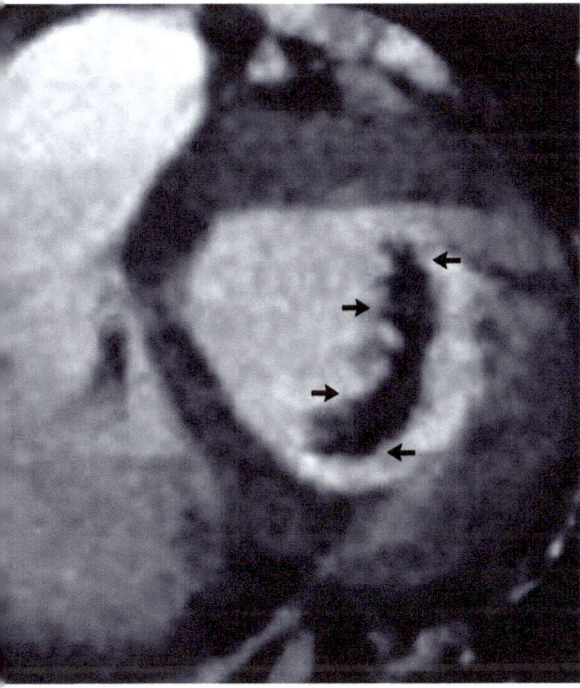

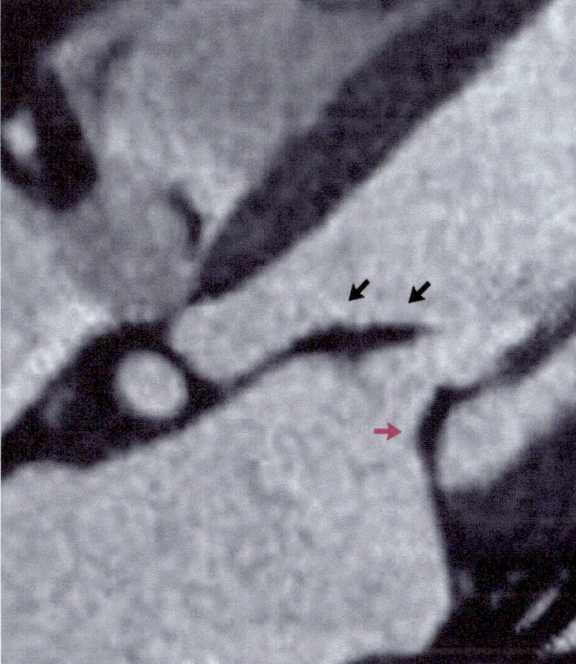

[3] Short axis view at the 10% R-R interval shows thickening of the mitral valve (arrows).

[4] 4-chamber view at the 60% R-R interval shows doming of the aortic valve (dark arrows) and limited motion of the posterior leaflet is seen (pink arrow).

Cardiac
Morphology

Foong Koon Cheah
John Huang

Department of Radiology
Singapore General Hospital
Singapore

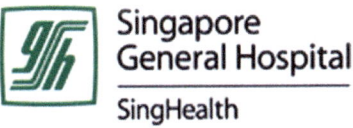

Cardiac
Morphology

Basic considerations

Accurate assessment of cardiac morphology is often facilitated by evaluation of the heart throughout the cardiac cycle. An ECG-pulsing window from 30–70% allows reconstruction of images in both systole and diastole. Scan coverage area is adapted depending on the indication. The entire chest should be imaged for the evaluation of congenital heart disease and cardiac masses.

Evaluation of both right- and left-sided cardiac chambers is optimized by homogeneous contrast enhancement throughout the heart. Therefore, the main contrast bolus is followed by a second bolus diluted with saline to a 30% concentration to maintain adequate cardiac enhancement while reducing artifacts from dense contrast in the SVC and brachiocephalic veins. [1]

Scan Parameters

Scan mode	Dual Source, ECG-gated
Heart rate control	not necessary
Scan area	heart or whole chest*
Scan direction	cranio-caudal
Scan time	~8 s, depending on heart rate*
Tube voltage	100 kV*
Tube current	360 mAs/rotation*
Dose modulation	CARE Dose4D, ECG-pulsing (details in Table on page 22)*
$CTDI_{vol}$	~40 mGy, depending on heart rate*
Rotation time	0.33 s
Pitch	0.2–0.5, depending on heart rate
Slice collimation	0.6 mm
Acquisition	64 x 0.6 mm
Slice width	0.75 mm
Reconstruction increment	0.4 mm
Reconstruction kernel	B26f

* **Asian Adaptation by Singapore General Hospital**
Due to the slimmer population in Asia, typically lower kV values at an adjusted quality ref. mAs/rot. level in combination with CARE Dose4D are used which leads to lower radiation exposure.

Tricks

If suspicious of pericardial disease or cardiac mass, perform non-contrast scan first to assess calcification and enhancement characteristics. For larger patients, consider increasing contrast injection rate. Cine loops in short axis and 4-chamber long axis (0–95%, every 5%) using 8 mm section width and 6 mm increment are viewed on every case. [1]

Pitfalls

If the duration of the contrast bolus is too short, the evaluation of cardiac morphology will be compromised, particularly of the right-sided cardiac chambers. Consider performing an additional venous-phase scan for the evaluation of pericardial inflammation or cardiac mass. [1]

Contrast Injection Protocol

	Iodine concentration 370 mg I/ml
Injection scheme	Monophasic
Iodine delivery rate	1.85 g/s
CM volume	5 ml/s for duration of scan plus 40 ml diluted to 30%
CM flow rate	5 ml/s
Body weight adaptation	yes
Bolus timing	bolus tracking **
Bolus tracking threshold	150 HU
ROI position	ascending aorta
Scan delay	4 s
Saline flush volume	60 ml
Saline injection rate	5 ml/s
Needle size	18 G
Injection site	antecubital vein

** Depending on the preference of the individual site, test bolus can be used as an alternative

[1] S. Harris, C. McCollough, E. Williamson in [1]

Case 1
Atrial Septal Defect (I)

Case history

A 44-year-old female presenting with chest discomfort and exertional dyspnoea was found to have a secundum atrial septal defect (ASD) with a deficient aortic rim on trans-oesophageal echocardiography. Cardiac CT was performed primarily to exclude coronary artery disease prior to surgical closure of the ASD.

Diagnosis/Differential diagnosis

An ASD was found. The coronary arteries were normal.

Findings

There was no evidence of coronary artery disease. The ASD was well visualized, along with concomitant dilatation of the right ventricle and flattening of the interventricular septum.

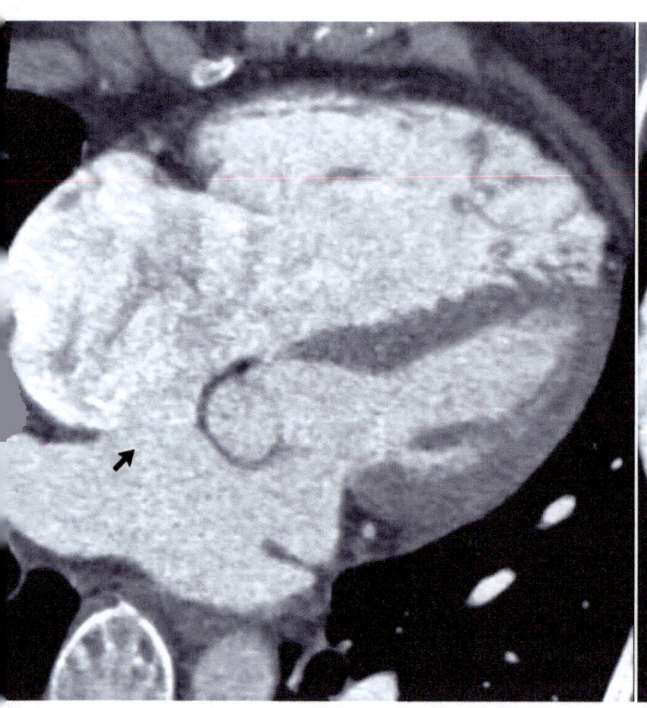
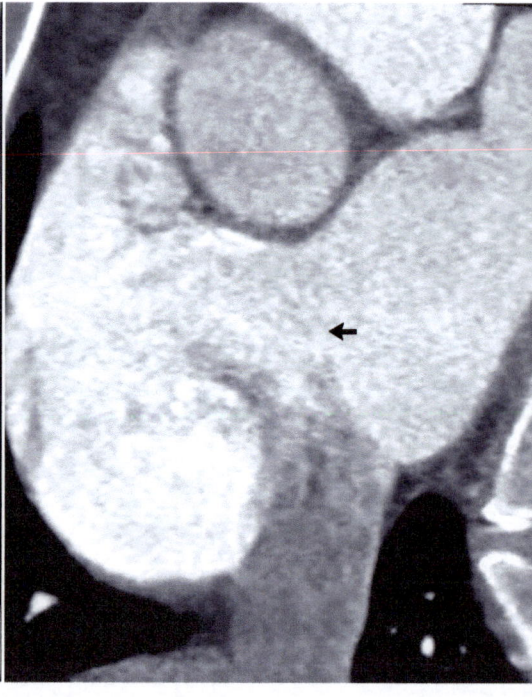

[1] Horizontal long axis multiplanar reformation (MPR) of the heart shows the ASD.

[2] Short axis MPR at the level of the atria demonstrates the ASD.

Take-home message

Cardiac morphology and congenital defects are well demonstrated by CT. The assessment of cardiac function is further aided by the improved temporal resolution of DSCT.

Optimal opacification of the cardiac chambers and vessels of interest can be challenging due to the presence of shunts and surgical bypass. We favor a test bolus approach to address this issue.

The use of a mixed saline/contrast flush is useful to help reduce streak artifacts from dense contrast in the SVC and right atrium.

Differential flow or unexpected opacification of certain cardiac or vascular structures should alert one to the presence of an underlying shunt.

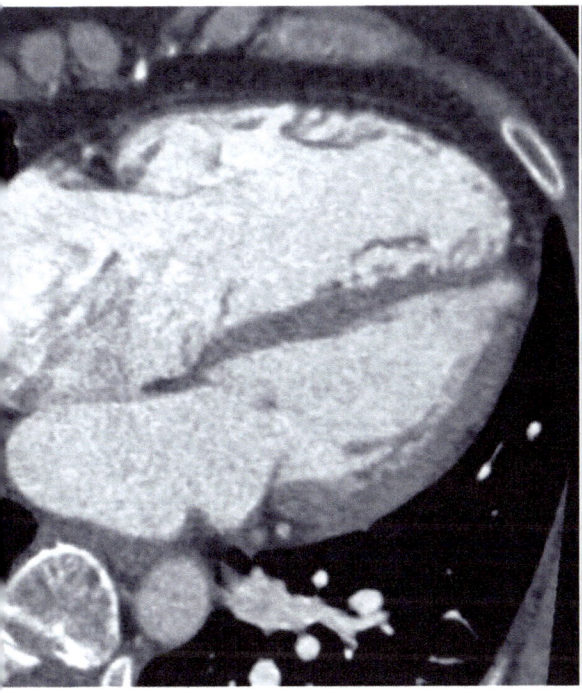 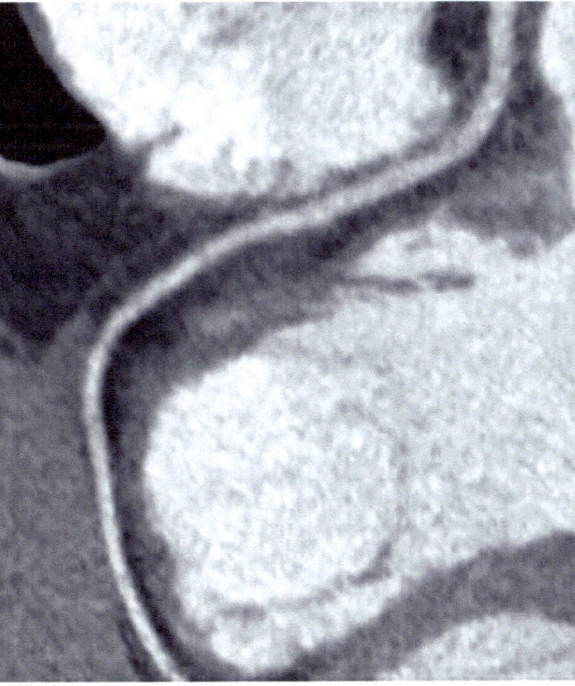

[3] Four-chamber view of the heart shows dilatation of the right ventricle with flattening of the interventricular septum.

[4] Curved MPR of the right coronary artery shows a vessel which is disease-free.

Case 2
Atrial Septal Defect (II)

Case history
A 42-year-old female presented with a history of pulmonary stenosis treated by pulmonary valvotomy many years ago. Now, a pulmonary regurgitation had occurred. Echocardiogram showed an unidentified flap-like structure in the right atrium.

Diagnosis / Differential diagnosis
There was a dilated pulmonary artery in keeping with the history of pulmonary stenosis, post pulmonary valvotomy. Sinus venosus showed ASD.

Findings
The main and left pulmonary arteries were dilated in keeping with the history of pulmonary stenosis. A defect was demonstrated in the sinus venosus part of the atrial septum, allowing contrast flow from the left atrium into the IVC. This was in keeping with a low sinus venosus type ASD.

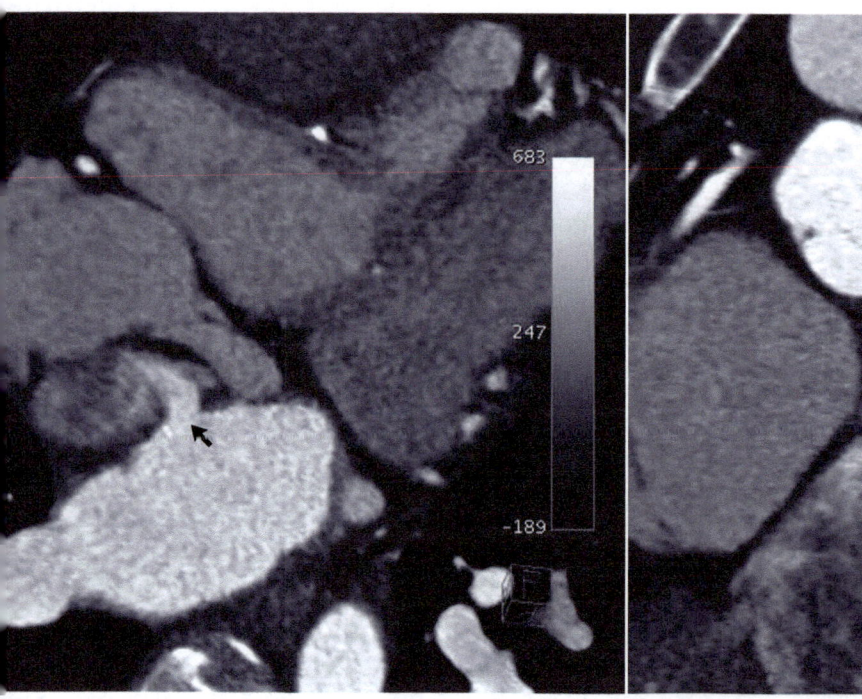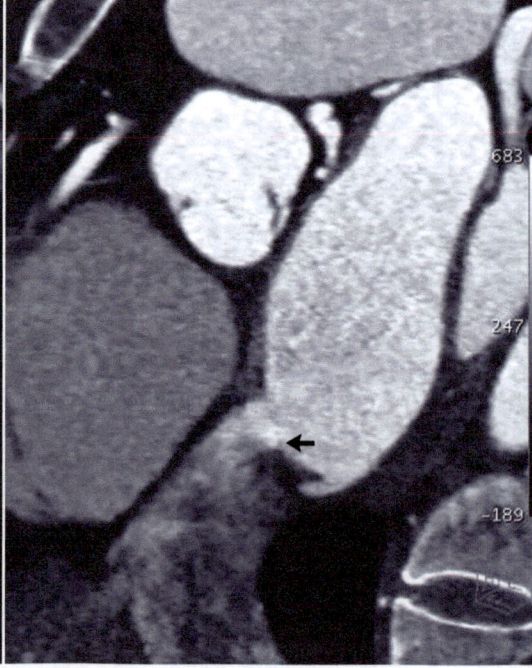

[1] Horizontal long axis view depicting the communication between the left atrium and IVC (arrow).

[2] Short axis view through the atria showing passage of contrast from the left atrium to IVC (arrow).

The right ventricular wall did not show overt hypertrophy.

Take-home message

Cardiac morphology and congenital defects are well demonstrated by CT. The assessment of cardiac function is further aided by the improved temporal resolution of DSCT.

Optimal opacification of the cardiac chambers and vessels of interest can be challenging in the presence of shunts and surgical bypasses. We favor a test bolus approach to address this issue. The use of a mixed saline/contrast flush is useful to help reduce streak artifacts from dense contrast in the SVC and right atrium.

Differential flow or unexpected opacification of certain cardiac or vascular structures should alert one to the presence of an underlying shunt.

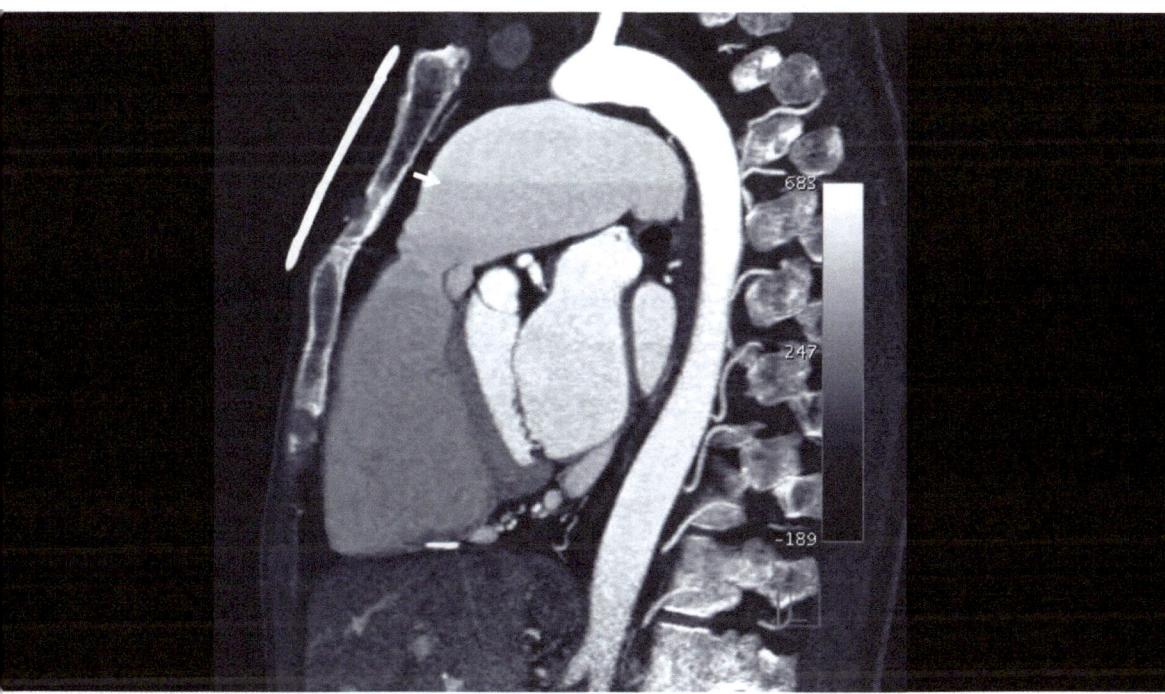

[3] Sagittal view of the dilated main pulmonary artery (arrow).

Cardiac
Atrial Fibrillation /
Arrhythmia

Song Lan
Wang Yining
Zhang Zhuhua
Kong Lingyan
Jin Zhengyu

Department of Radiology
Peking Union Medical College Hospital
Beijing, China

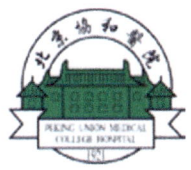

Cardiac
Atrial Fibrillation/Arrhythmia

Basic considerations

The presence of atrial fibrillation requires a fixed, low pitch (generally 0.2) irrespective of baseline heart rate, because the heart rate may vary significantly throughout the scan.
If a relatively fast pitch is selected, e.g. in patients with a high baseline heart rate during the last 10 beats prior to the start of the scan, extensive interpolation artifacts will occur if the heart rate drops more than 10 bpm during the scan. A multi-segment reconstruction algorithm should not be used in patients with arrhythmia, because the data of two consecutive heart beats at a different contraction phase will be merged, resulting in poor image quality due to blurring. [1]

Scan Parameters

Scan mode	Dual Source, ECG-gated
Heart rate control	not necessary
Scan area	mid pulmonary artery to below heart
Scan direction	cranio-caudal
Scan time	~11–12 s, depending on heart rate*
Tube voltage	120 kV
Tube current	360 mAs/rotation
Dose modulation	ECG-pulsing on, 25–70%
$CTDI_{vol}$	~45–60 mGy, depending on heart rate*
Rotation time	0.33 s
Pitch	0.2 (fixed)
Slice collimation	0.6 mm
Acquisition	64 x 0.6 mm
Slice width	0.75 mm
Reconstruction increment	0.4 mm
Reconstruction kernel	B26f, B46f in case of excessive calcification

* Asian Adaptation by PUMC, Beijing

Tricks

Carefully check the position of the reconstruction windows in every heart beat to avoid step artifacts. Edit reconstruction windows positioned in arrhythmic heart beats, if possible. End-systolic datasets generally provide optimal image quality, because this interval is relatively constant even in arrhythmic heart beats. [1]

Pitfalls

A percentage reconstruction algorithm is very sensitive to arrhythmia and should therefore not be used in patients with atrial fibrillation. Absolute forward reconstruction (fixed delay after R-peak in ms) is especially useful to obtain end-systolic datasets, which is often the best phase in patients with arrhythmia, especially if the baseline heart rate is high. [1]

Contrast Injection Protocol

	Iodine concentration 370 mg I/ml
Injection scheme	Monophasic
Iodine delivery rate	1.85 g/s
CM volume	5 ml/s for duration of scan, ≥ 50 ml
CM flow rate	5 ml/s
Body weight adaptation	no
Bolus timing	bolus tracking **
Bolus tracking threshold	100 HU
ROI position	ascending aorta
Scan delay	peak time plus 2 s
Saline flush volume	60 ml
Saline injection rate	5 ml/s
Needle size	18 G
Injection site	antecubital vein

** Depending on the preference of the individual site, test bolus can be used as an alternative

[1] N. Mollet, F. Cademartiri, G. Krestin in [1]

Case 1
Atrial Fibrillation and Acute Chest Pain

Case history

A 73-year-old female presented with new onset of atypical chest pain. The ECG of the patient showed atrial fibrillation. She had hypertension and diabetes.

Diagnosis / Differential diagnosis

Mild calcification was detected. Significant stenosis was observed in the proximal segment of LAD and Diag1 arteries accompanied with atherosclerotic plaque. Calcified plaque was detected in the middle RCA, but without significant stenoses.

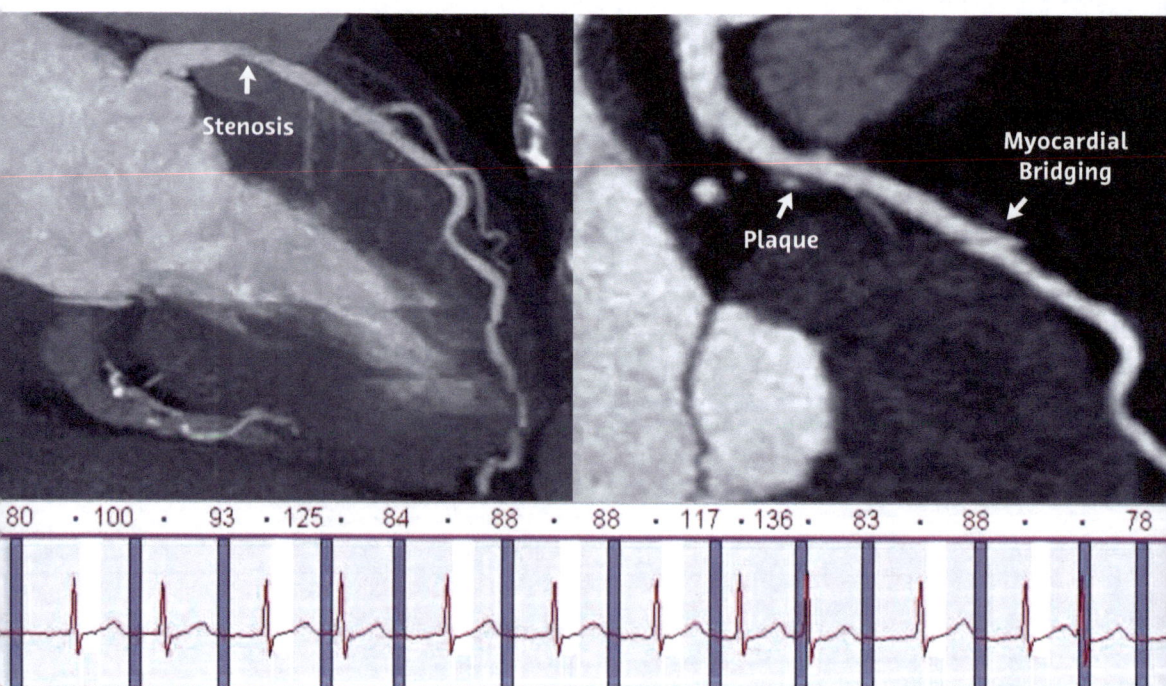

MIP and CPR images of coronary CT angiography show significant proximal LAD and Diag1 stenosis. Cross-sectional images of the stenosis show large predominantly non-calcified plaques.

Curved MPR image of LAD indicates a myocardial bridging located at middle LAD and the absence of significant coronary stenoses, despite the presence of residual step artifacts.

Findings

There was an atrial fibrillation rhythm, heart rate during acquisition was 93 bpm (71–171 bpm). An end-systolic dataset (reconstructed +225 ms after the previous R-wave) provided optimal image quality. Except for the LAD and Diag1 stenosis, additional significant coronary stenoses could reliably be ruled out despite the presence of several step artifacts located at the distal segment of LAD.

Take-home message

The percentage approach is more sensitive to arrhythmia when compared to absolute forward or backward reconstruction phase selection. End-systolic datasets frequently provide optimal image quality in patients with arrhythmia, especially when the heart rate is relatively high (above 70 bpm). It may not be possible to completely diminish all step artifacts; however, stenosis detection is generally not significantly affected by these artifacts.

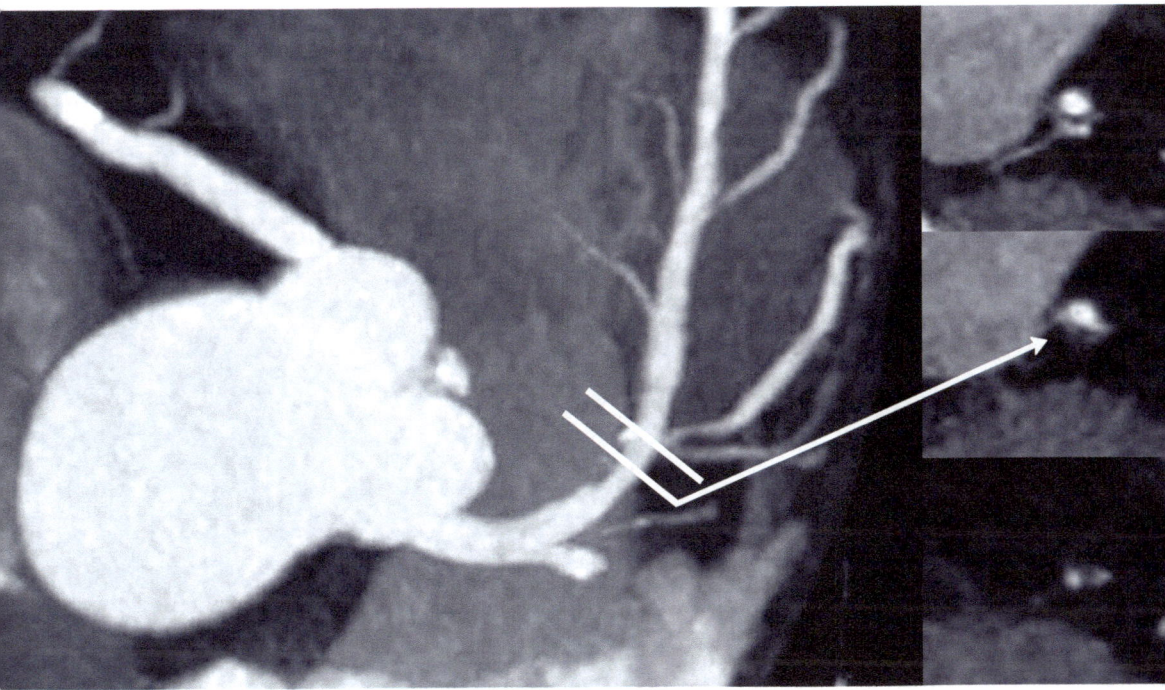

Case 2
Atrial Fibrillation and Chronic Chest Pain

Case history

A 59-year-old female presented with chest pain and palpitation for about 10 years. The ECG of the patient showed atrial fibrillation. She had neither hypertension nor diabetes.

Diagnosis / Differential diagnosis

There was no evidence of coronary artery disease disease). Cardiac structure and function were normal, with no CT evidence of valvular abnormalities. Non-cardiac structures were unremarkable.

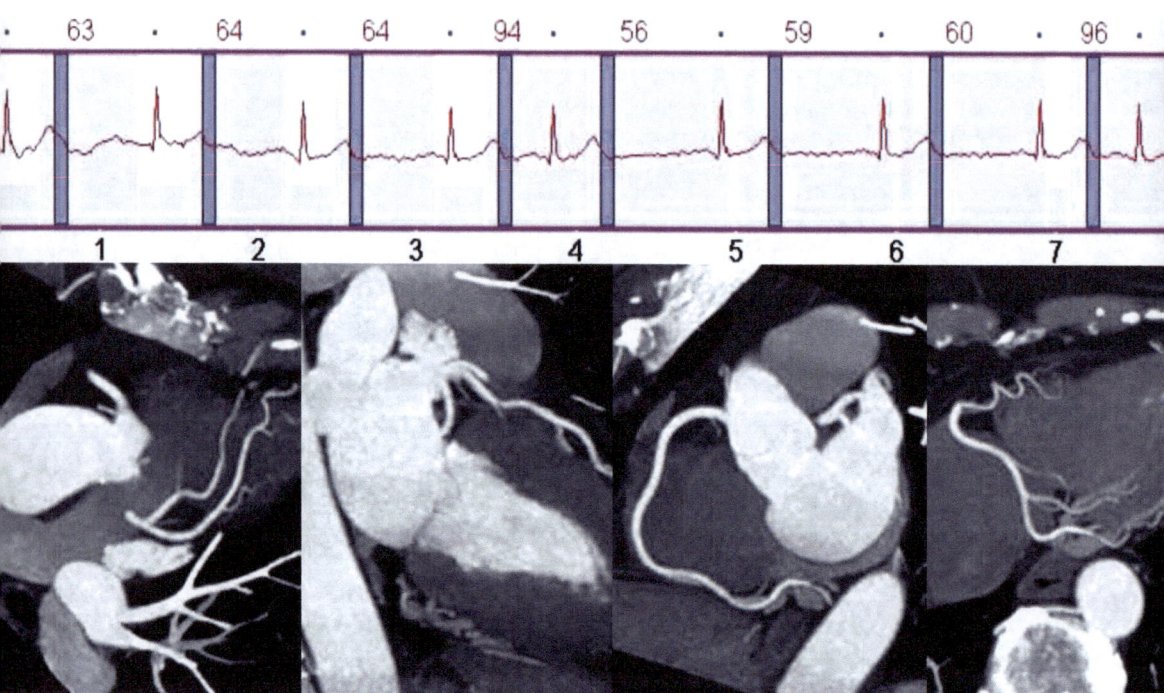

Despite the ECG showing atrial fibrillation, no evidence of coronary artery disease and no CT evidence of valvular abnormalities were found.

Findings

There was an atrial fibrillation rhythm, heart rate during acquisition was 66 bpm (56 – 96 bpm). An end-systolic dataset (reconstructed +300 ms after the previous R-wave) provided optimal image quality. All artery segments were well shown without any motion artifact.

Take-home message

The percentage approach is more sensitive to arrhythmia compared to the ms approach. End-systolic datasets frequently provide optimal image quality in patients with arrhythmia, especially when the heart rate is relatively high (above 70 bpm).

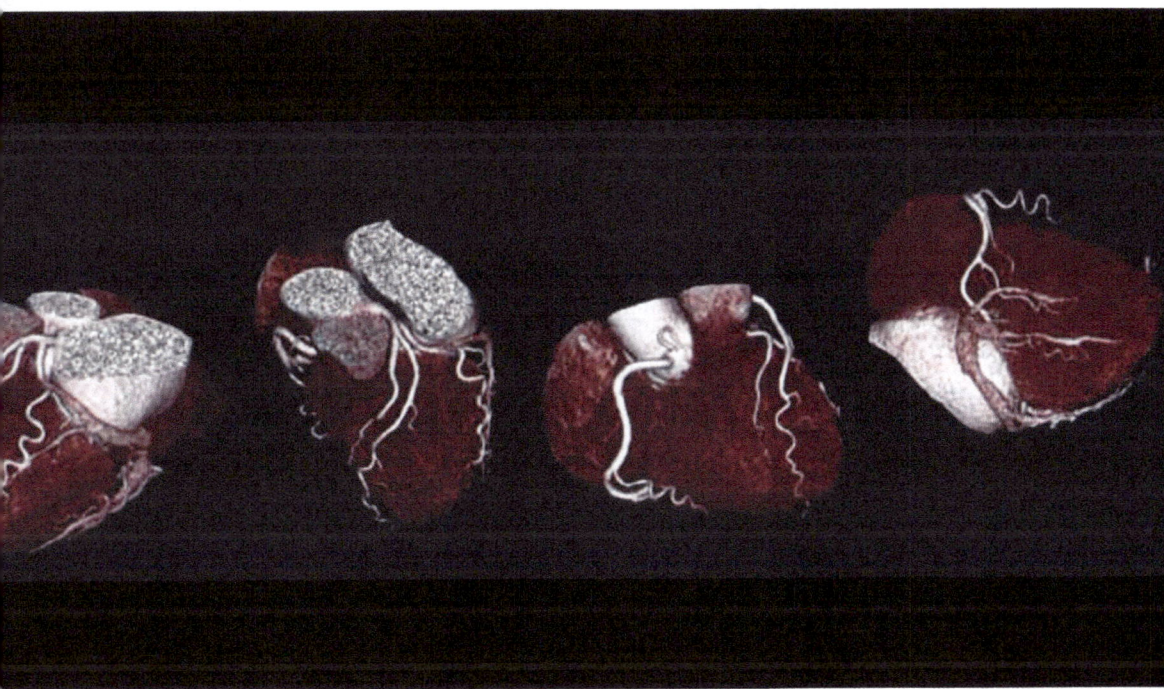

Volume-rendered images show no occlusions.

Cardiac
Bypass Grafts

Gongyong Jin
Youngkon Kim
Hyosung Kwak

Department of Radiology
Chonbuk National University Hospital
Jeonju, Republic of Korea

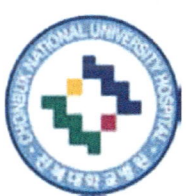

Cardiac
Bypass Grafts

Basic considerations

No calcium-scoring needed because there is established coronary disease. Scan entire chest from above the clavicles through the diaphragm to include the entire IMA if bypass situation is unknown or if there is a known IMA graft. Start at the aortic arch if only venous grafts are present. ECG-pulsing should be used to reduce radiation exposure. Use MinDose™ if functional information is not of concern. If myocardial hypoattenuation is seen upon coronary CTA, consider acquiring a thick section (1.2 mm collimation) low kV (80 or 100 kV) scan for delayed enhancement and viability assessment. [1]

Scan Parameters

Scan mode	Dual Source, ECG-gated
Heart rate control	not necessary
Scan area	clavicle (or arch) to diaphragm
Scan direction	cranio-caudal
Scan time	~15 – 16 s, depending on heart rate *
Tube voltage	100 kV *
Tube current	360 mAs/rotation
Dose modulation	ECG-pulsing (details in Table on page 22)
CTDI$_{vol}$	~40 mGy, depending on heart rate *
Rotation time	0.33 s
Pitch	0.2 0.5, depending on heart rate
Slice collimation	0.6 mm
Acquisition	64 x 0.6 mm
Slice width	0.75 mm *
Reconstruction increment	0.4 mm *
Reconstruction kernel	B26f *

* Asian Adaptation by Chonbuk National University Hospital
Due to the slimmer population in Asia, typically lower kV values at an adjusted mAs/rot. level are used which leads to lower CTDI$_{vol}$ values.

Tricks

Increase mAs in obese patients. Use smoother kernels (B20f) and thicker sections for obese patients. Use sharper kernel (B46f) for reconstruction in patients with stents and/or heavy calcifications. Start with 3D (VRT) view to understand overall graft anatomy, then review MPRs and curved MPRs. [1]

Pitfalls

Automatic segmentation of heart may remove some of the bypass grafts. Shell-like circumferential calcifications may look like stents. Inappropriate windowing may make it difficult to differentiate vessel lumen filled with high attenuation contrast media from calcifications. Preferably, use right arm for IV, to avoid proximal left IMA being obscured by streaks. [1]

Contrast Injection Protocol

	Iodine concentration 370 mg I/ml
Injection scheme	Monophasic
Iodine delivery rate	1.85 g/s
CM volume	5 ml/s for duration of scan, ≥ 50 ml
CM flow rate	5 ml/s
Body weight adaptation	no
Bolus timing	test bolus **
Bolus tracking threshold	n.a.
ROI position	ascending aorta
Scan delay	test bolus peak time
Saline flush volume	60 ml of CM/Saline (30/70%)
Saline injection rate	5 ml/s
Needle size	18 G
Injection site	right antecubital vein

** Depending on the preference of the individual site, bolus tracking can be used as an alternative

[1] P. Suranyi, C. Thilo, H. Lee, U.J. Schoepf in [1]

Case 1
Acute Graft Occlusion (I)

Case history

This 72-year-old male was admitted in our hospital due to a mild dyspnea for several days. He had undergone CABG in our institution 3 months before.

What is the cause of the mild dyspnea? Are any of the bypass grafts occluded/stenotic, or is the cause of the dyspnea extra-cardiac?

Diagnosis / Differential diagnosis

Total occlusion of two saphenous venous grafts was due to the acute graft thrombosis.

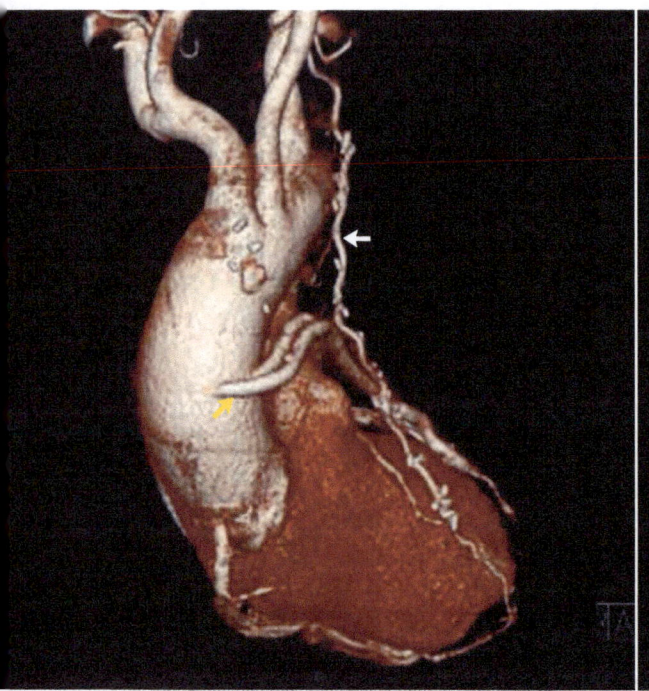

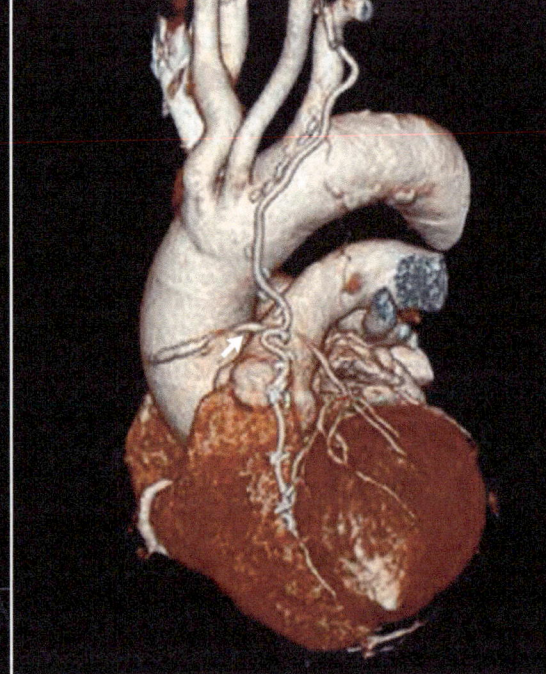

[1] 3D volume-rendering of CABG. There was good patency at left IMA-LAD (white arrow), SVG from aorta-PDA of RCA, and SVG from aorta-1st OM of LCX (yellow arrow).

[2] 3D volume-rendering of CABG. Three months later, SVG from aorta-PDA of RCA was totally occluded and SVG from aorta-1st OM of LCX was almost totally occluded (white arrow).

Findings

Although the left IMA appeared patent, there was a severe stenosis (to the first obtuse marginal branch (OM1) of LCX) or total occlusion (to posterior descending artery of RCA) at two venous grafts. On invasive coronary angiography, the same results showed.

Take-home message

In patients with persistent dyspnea of unknown origin following CABG surgery, coronary CTA is an excellent tool for differential diagnosis. Acute graft occlusion can be quickly and efficiently diagnosed with Dual Source CT, while additional valuable information is also gained about the chest wall, lungs, other thoracic vessels, and the native coronary arteries.

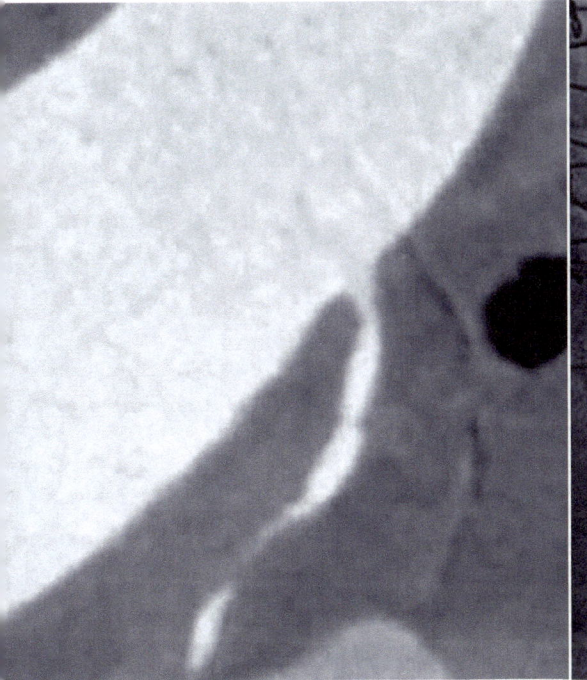

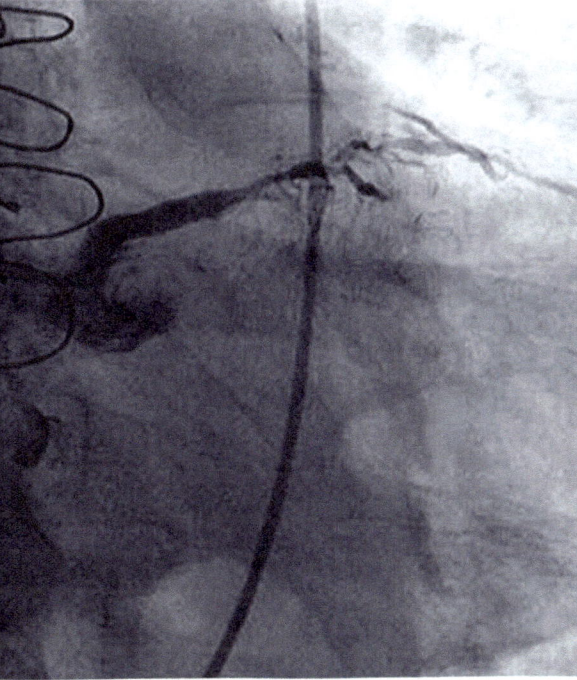

[3] Curved MPR of the venous graft, proximal portion from aorta showed severe stenosis/total occlusion.

[4] On invasive coronary angiography, findings of total occluded graft showed the same results as compared to coronary CT angiography. There was nearly total occlusion at SVG from aorta-1st OM of LCX.

Case 2
Acute Graft Occlusion (II)

Case history

This 57-year-old female complained of chest pain for several days. She had undergone CABG operation eight months before.

What is the cause of the chest pain? Are any of the acute bypass grafts occluded/stenotic, or is the cause of the dyspnea and chest pain extra-cardiac?

Diagnosis / Differential diagnosis

Acute graft thrombosis was detected. D/Dx. pericarditis, acute pulmonary thromboembolism were also observed.

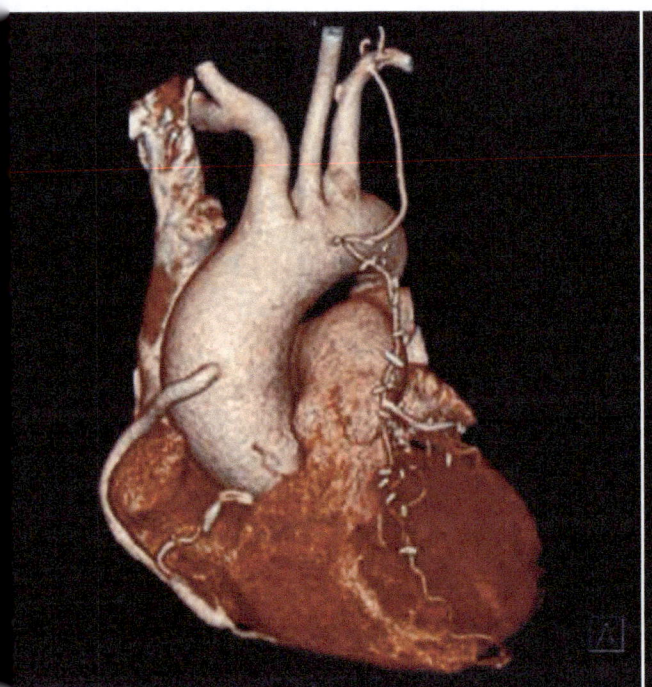 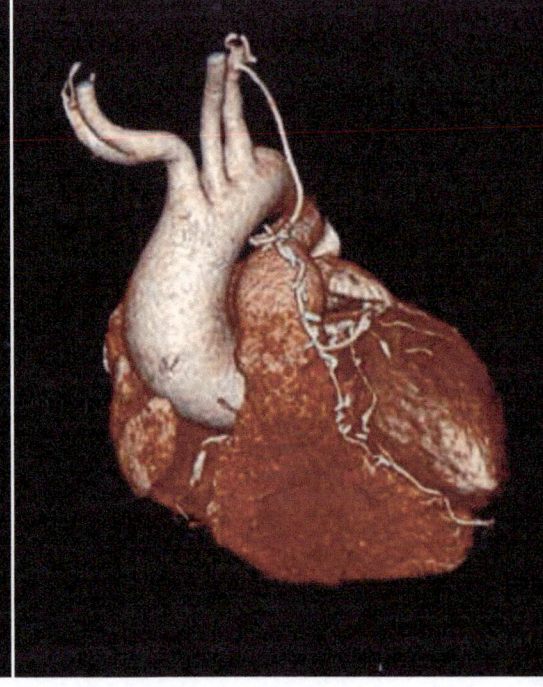

[1] 3D volume-rendering of CABG, the left IMA and venous graft was intact at post-operation follow-up CT.

[2] 3D volume-rendering of CABG, although the left IMA was intact but venous graft from aorta was totally occluded on 8 months follow-up CT.

Findings

Although the left IMA was intact, venous graft (SVG from aorta – PDA of RCA) showed total occlusion at the origination of the ascending aorta. On invasive angiography, the venous graft at the origination of the ascending aorta was totally occluded. After balloon dilatation at the stenotic site of the venous graft and stent insertion were performed, normal venous graft showed on invasive coronary angiography.

Take-home message

In patients with persistent dyspnea of unknown origin following CABG surgery, coronary CTA is an excellent tool for differential diagnosis. The absence of acute graft occlusion can be quickly and efficiently diagnosed with Dual Source CT, while additional valuable information is also gained about acute pneumonia, acceleration of bronchial asthma, pericardial effusion, etc.

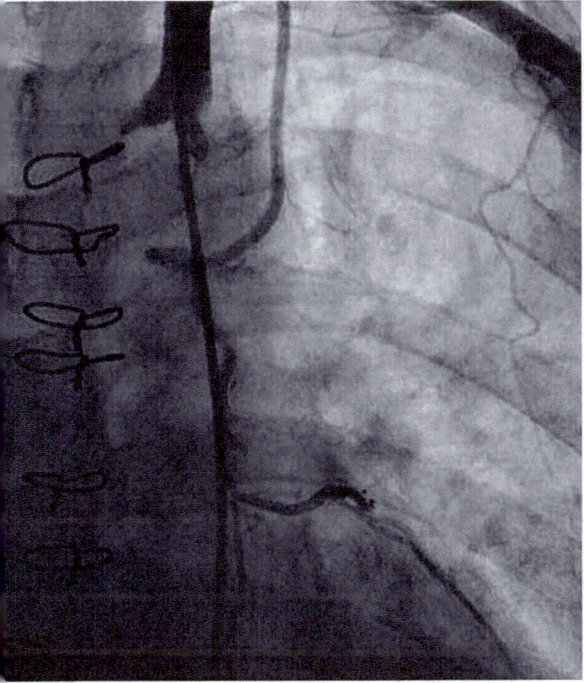

[3] On invasive coronary angiography, venous graft was totally occluded.

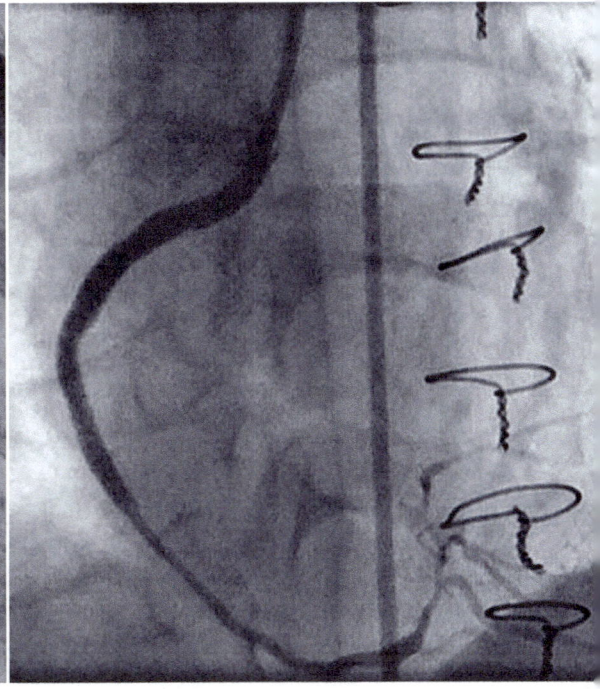

[4] After stent inserted into the stenotic venous graft, normalized venous graft showed on invasive coronary angiography.

Vascular
Extended Chest Pain Protocol

Kwang Nam Jin
Eun-Ah Park
Whal Lee

Department of Radiology
Seoul National University Hospital
Seoul, Korea

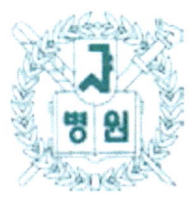
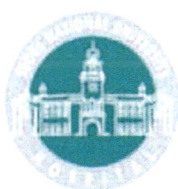

Vascular
Extended Chest Pain Protocol

Basic considerations

There are some important technical aspects to consider in extended chest pain protocol. First, the scan range is larger, causing longer scan time, increase in volume of contrast media, and additional radiation exposure. Second, it is very challenging to obtain consistent and high enhancement of all three vascular beds. A dedicated contrast media protocol is necessary. With a relatively low threshold of 80 HU above which the scan was initiated, homogeneous attenuation in the aortic, coronary and pulmonary arteries could be achieved. By doing so, the time interval where the contrast enhancement curve of the pulmonary circulation overlaps with the enhancement of the aorta could be obtained. Last, caudo-cranial scan direction can avoid motion artifact of the basal lung, which mimics pulmonary thromboembolism, by scanning the basal lung earlier.

Scan Parameters

Scan mode	Dual Source, ECG-gated
Heart rate control	not necessary
Scan area	diaphragm to lung apex
Scan direction	caudo-cranial
Scan time	~12–20 s, depending on heart rate
Tube voltage	100 kV
Tube current	360 mAs / rotation
Dose modulation	ECG-pulsing with MinDose™ (details in Table on page 22)
$CTDI_{vol}$	~35 mGy, depending on heart rate
Rotation time	0.33 s
Pitch	0.2–0.5, depending on heart rate
Slice collimation	0.6 mm
Acquisition	64 x 0.6 mm
Slice width	3 mm / 0.75 mm for coronary arteries
Reconstruction increment	2 mm / 0.4 mm
Reconstruction kernel	B26f

Asian Adaptation by Seoul National University Hospital
Due to the slimmer population in Asia, typically lower kV values at an adjusted mAs/rot. level are used which leads to lower $CTDI_{vol}$ values.

Tricks

Plan the range precisely from the diaphragm to the lung apex to limit radiation exposure. Do not instruct patients to take a deep breath, but just to hold their breath after mild inspiration. Reconstruct thin slices with a limited FoV of the heart to provide sufficient detail and a stack of 3 mm images for assessment of the chest.

Pitfalls

Fast and deep inspiration can interrupt the contrast bolus due to inflow of non-enhanced blood from the inferior vena cava, often causing insufficient pulmonary opacification.

Contrast Injection Protocol

	Iodine concentration 370 mg I/ml
Injection scheme	Monophasic
Iodine delivery rate	1.7 g/s
CM volume	100 ml
CM flow rate	4.5 ml/s
Body weight adaptation	yes
Bolus timing	bolus tracking **
Bolus tracking threshold	80 HU
ROI position	ascending aorta
Scan delay	6 s
Saline flush volume	60 ml
Saline injection rate	4.5 ml/s
Needle size	18 G
Injection site	antecubital vein

** Depending on the preference of the individual site, test bolus can be used as an alternative

Case 1
59-year-old Male with Typical Chest Pain

Case history

A 59-year-old male, current smoker, was admitted to our hospital due to typical chest pain while at rest. He had experienced similar chest pain twice before. He showed no response to nitroglycerin. He had been treated with anti-hypertensive medication. At admission, initial ECG was normal. Initial Troponin I and CKMB levels were 0.35 ng/mL (0~0.5) and 2.2 ng/mL (0.6~6.3).

Diagnosis / Differential diagnosis

Non-ST elevation myocardial infarction was clinically suspected. Other cardiovascular causes for acute chest pain, including aortic dissection or pulmonary embolism, needed to be ruled out.

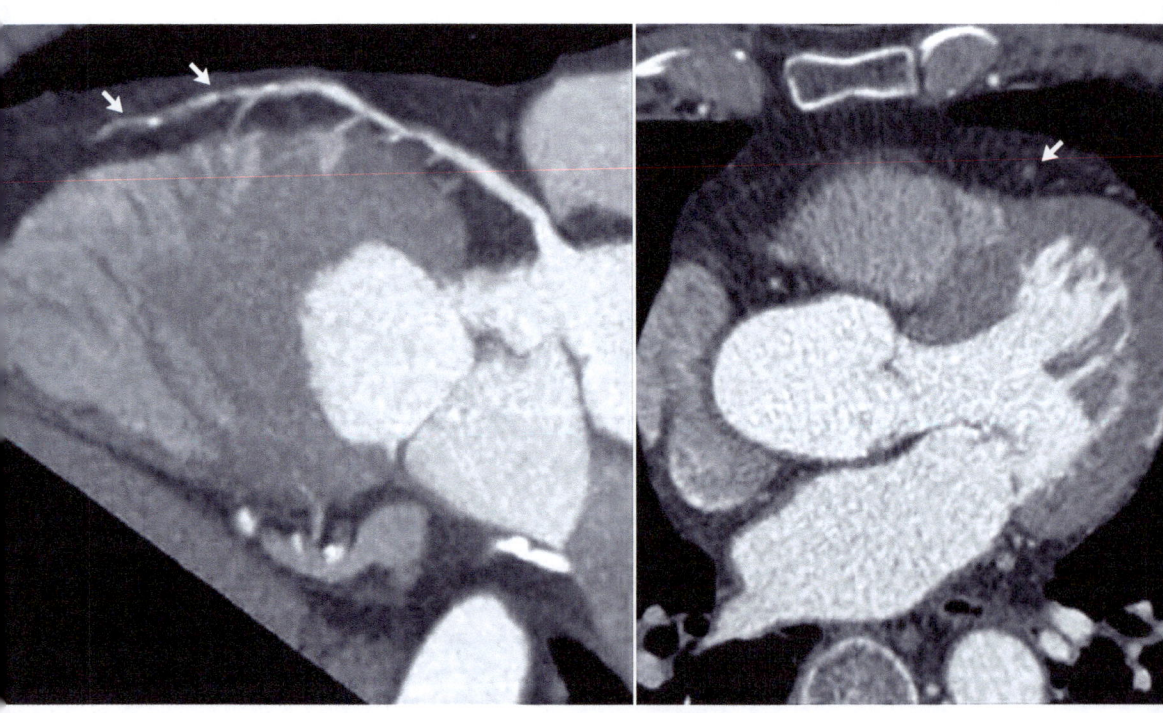

[1] Curved multiplanar reconstruction (MPR) image shows multiple significant stenosis in the distal left anterior descending (LAD) coronary artery (arrows).

[2] No enhancement of distal LAD is seen on axial image (arrow).

Findings

CT images revealed no enhancement of distal left anterior descending coronary artery and hypo-enhancement of corresponding myocardial territory, suggestive of acute myocardial infarction. In addition, chronic total occlusion in the distal left circumflex artery and obtuse marginal branch was shown. On follow-up ECG, T wave inversion at V2-4 developed. Troponin I and CKMB levels were also elevated.

Take-home message

Careful attention should be paid to myocardial enhancement in acute chest pain and a culprit lesion for the chest pain should be identified.

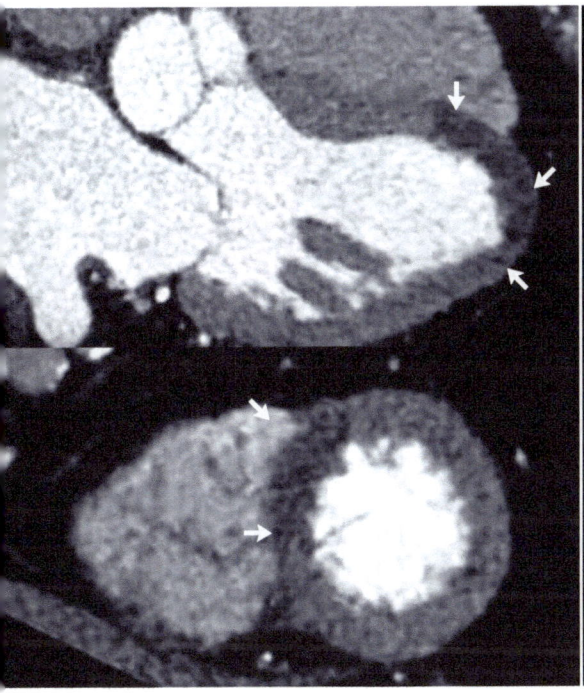

[3] MPR image shows hypoattenuation of mid to apical septal wall, suggestive of acute myocardial infarction of distal LAD territory (arrows).

[4] Volume-rendering image demonstrates nearly total occlusion in the proximal obtuse marginal branch (white arrow). Chronic total occlusion in the distal left circumflex artery is also noted (black arrow).

Case 2
Ruling out Cardiovascular Causes

Case history

A 70-year-old male smoker who was on medication for high blood pressure was admitted to our hospital due to unclear chest pain. Systolic blood pressure was 120 mm/Hg. Total cholesterol and HDL cholesterol levels were 188 mg/dL and 67 mg/dL. Pretest probability for CAD was high. Framingham risk score was 10%. The 10-year absolute risk of cardiac events of the patient was moderate. Troponin and ECG levels were within normal range.

Diagnosis / Differential diagnosis

Cardiovascular causes in acute chest pain, such as coronary artery disease, acute aortic dissection, and pulmonary thromboembolism, should be included as a differential diagnosis,

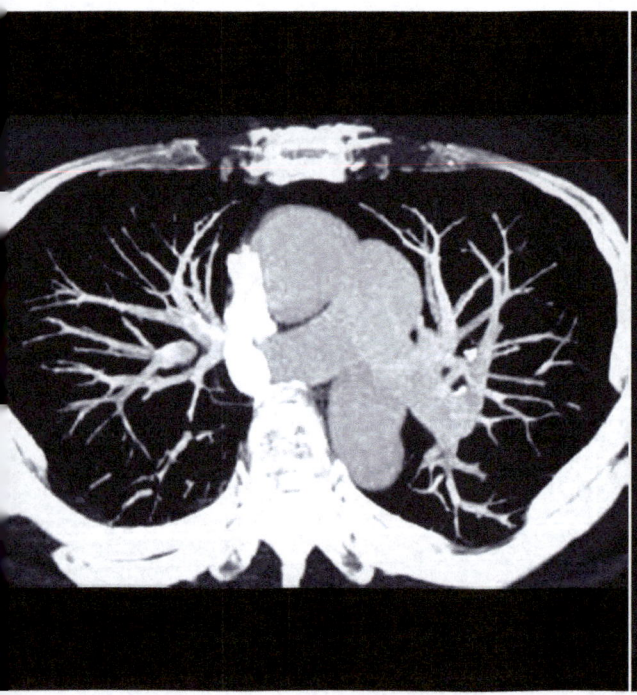
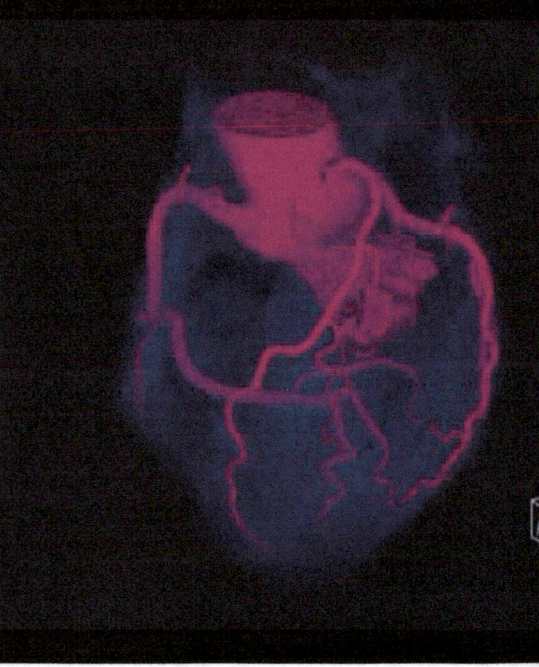

[1] Maximum intensity projection (MIP) axial image demonstrates normal pulmonary vessels. There is no intraluminal filling defect in both pulmonary arteries.

[2] Volume-rendering image demonstrates normal coronary arteries.

while pneumothorax and pneumonia should be excluded. Therefore, CT was performed to rule out cardiovascular causes in this patient with acute unclear chest pain.

Findings

There was no evidence of pulmonary embolism or aortic dissection. Coronary arteries were normal. However, global wall thickening of the apical segment was noted, suggestive of apical hypertrophic cardiomyopathy. To correlate the symptoms, a perfusion study such as myocardial SPECT or MRI with stress perfusion is recommended.

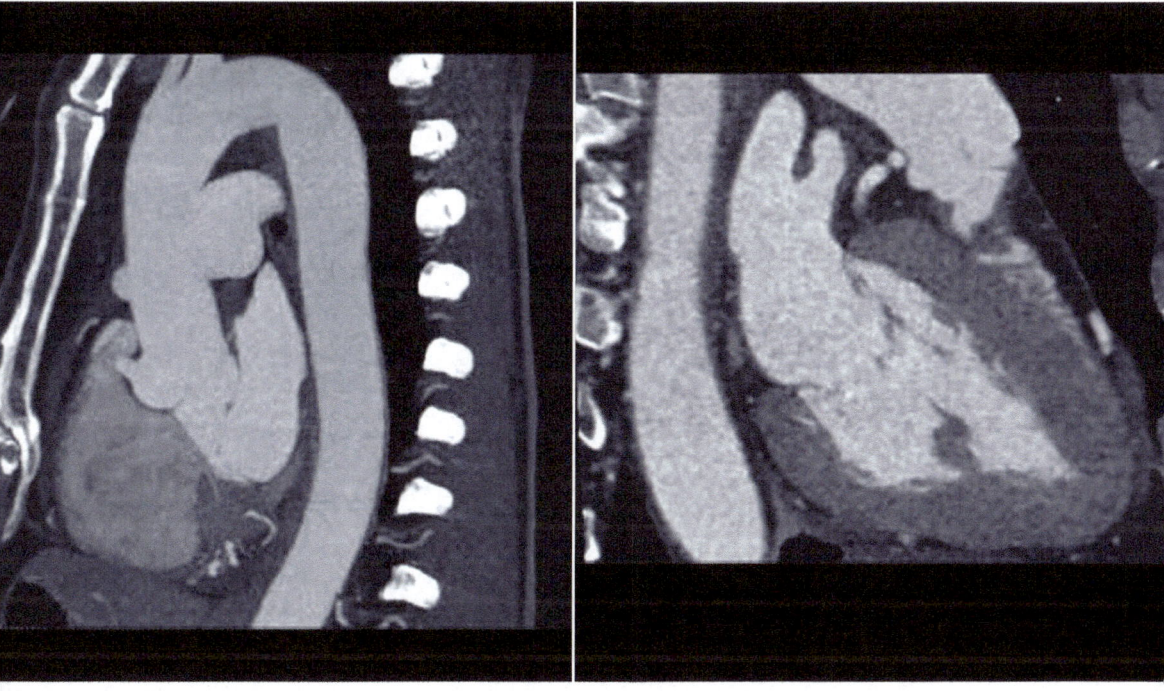

[3] Image shows normal thoracic aorta.

[4] Two-chamber view MPR image shows global wall thickening of the left ventricular apical segment, suggestive of apical hypertrophic cardiomyopathy.

Vascular
Pulmonary Veins

Dan Han
Lan Yan
Hui Duan

Imaging Centre
Kunming Medical College
Kunming, Yunnan, China

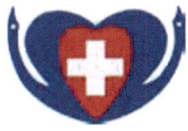

Vascular
Pulmonary Veins

Basic considerations

Although one would assume that the examination of pulmonary veins is fairly straightforward and easy, excellent images including 5th degree branches without any pulmonary artery opacification depend on the proper amount and injection rate of contrast agent given to the patients. Two scanning techniques are ECG-gated and non-gated single source mode, retrospectively. The examination may primarily be performed in a non-gated single source mode out of consideration for radiation dose. 100 kV/120 – 150 mAs may be considered in patients with low body mass index (BMI < 30).

Scan Parameters

Scan mode	Single Source, non-gated
Heart rate control	not necessary
Scan area	aortic arch to diaphragm*
Scan direction	caudo-cranial*
Scan time	~5 s
Tube voltage	100 kV
Tube current	200 quality ref. mAs*
Dose modulation	CARE Dose4D
CTDI$_{vol}$	~10 mGy
Rotation time	0.5 s*
Pitch	1
Slice collimation	0.6 mm
Acquisition	64 x 0.6 mm
Slice width	0.75 mm*
Reconstruction increment	0.5 mm*
Reconstruction kernel	B30f

* **Asian Adaptation by Kunming Medical College**
Higher image quality leads to slightly increased values for Quality ref. mAs, but due to the slimmer population in Asia, this still results in lower radiation exposure.

Tricks

Retrospectively ECG-gated mode should be reserved for patients with severe tachycardia and sinus-rhythm or regular conduction. With highly irregular conduction, non-gated scanning should be preferred irrespective of patients' heart rate.

Pitfalls

In principle, both bolus tracking or test bolus may be used for timing of the contrast injection. However, in case of irregular heart beat, cardiac output may change rapidly and test bolus procedure may provide insufficient results. In addition, for patients with higher body weight (> 90 kg), the test bolus might not reach a certain peak. Therefore, we suggest using bolus tracking in these patients.

Contrast Injection Protocol

	Iodine concentration 370 mg I/ml
Injection scheme	Monophasic
Iodine delivery rate	1.48 g/s
CM volume	60 ml*
CM flow rate	4 ml/s
Body weight adaptation	no
Bolus timing	bolus tracking**
Bolus tracking threshold	120 HU*
ROI position	left atrium
Scan delay	6 s*
Saline flush volume	60 ml
Saline injection rate	3 ml/s*
Needle size	18 G
Injection site	antecubital vein

** Depending on the preference of the individual site, test bolus can be used as an alternative

Case 1
A Type of Anatomical Mutations of Pulmonary Veins – Separate Ostium

Case history

A 51-year-old female had experienced a 3-year history of AF. CT reconstructions of left atrium and pulmonary veins were performed prior to RFCA.

Diagnosis/Differential diagnosis

Only one branch of right pulmonary venous drainage to the left atrium was detected. Atrial thrombi could be excluded.

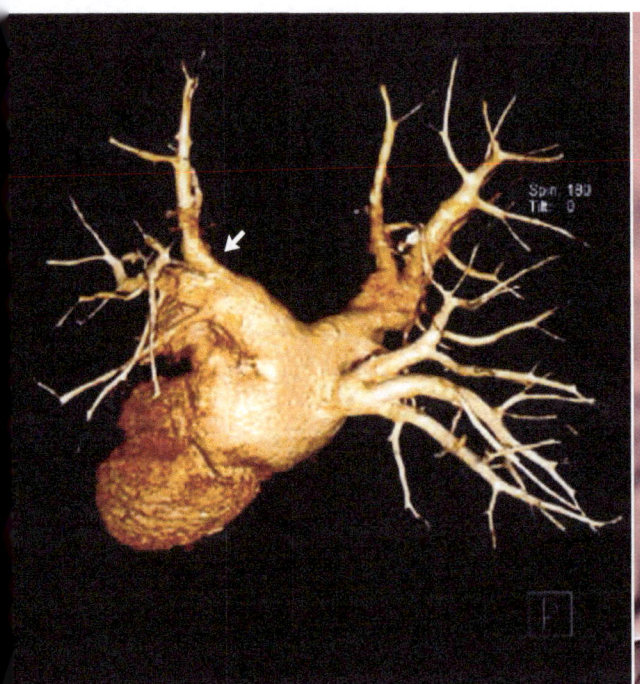

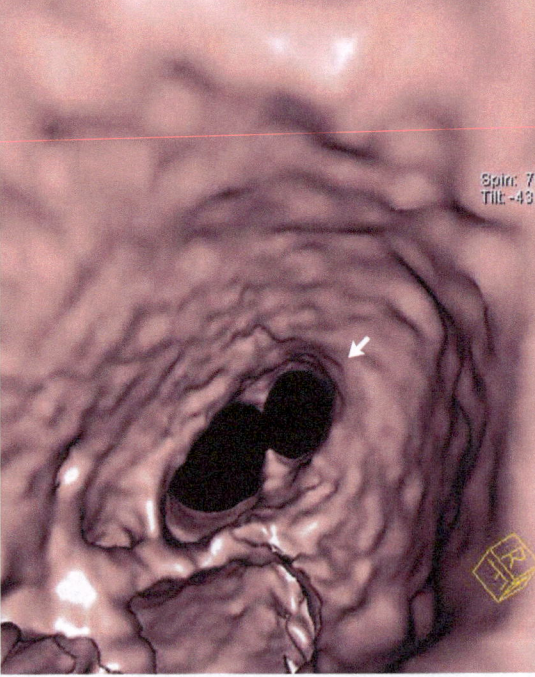

[1] VRT shows the only right upper pulmonary venous drainage to the left atrium in one-ostium format (arrow). Measurements can be performed by changing angles besides showing pulmonary venous drainage in VRT.

[2] VE shows the right pulmonary venous drainage to the left atrium in one-ostium format. Two ostia belong to the right upper pulmonary veins (arrow).

Findings

VRTs revealed separate ostia for upper, middle pulmonary venous on the right side and a branch drainage to the left atrium besides the main right lower pulmonary vein.

VE has verified that the left pulmonary vein had two ostia and the right pulmonary vein had four ostia which was a physiological variation.

Take-home message

Excellent image quality produced by DSCT can exactly demonstrate the anatomy of left atrium and pulmonary veins, provide useful morphological and anatomical information. Furthermore, the technology can be a non-invasive examination of AF and quantitatively analyze the data of patients for RFCA.

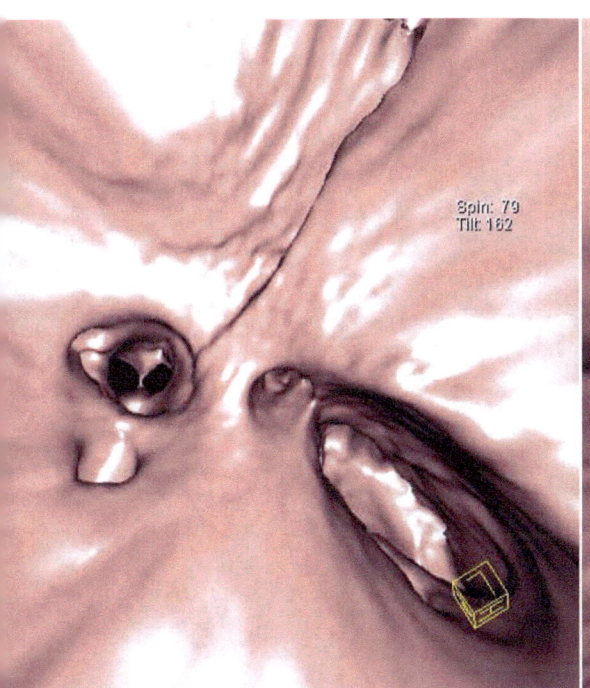

[3] VE shows the right pulmonary venous drainage to the left atrium in four-ostium format.

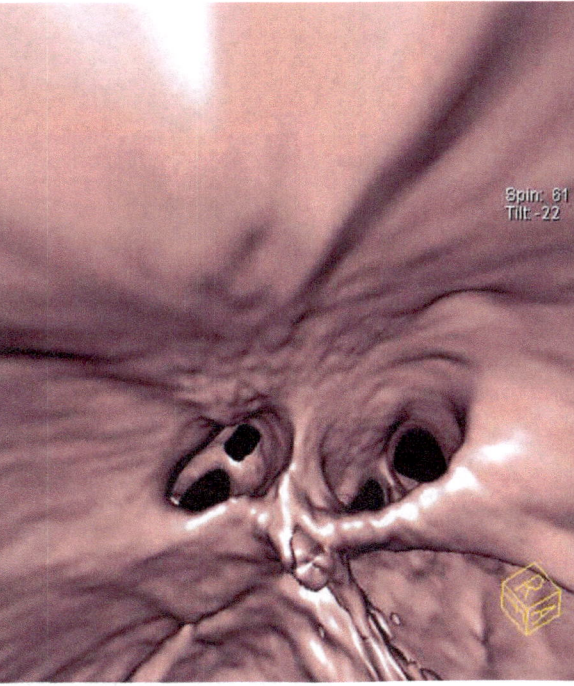

[4] VE shows the left pulmonary venous drainage to the left atrium in two-ostium format.

Case 2
A Type of Anatomical Mutations of Pulmonary Veins – Four Ostia

Case history

A 48-year-old male had a 3-year history of AF. CT reconstructions of left atrium and pulmonary veins were performed prior to RFCA.

Diagnosis/Differential diagnosis

Separate ostium for the right middle lobe vein was detected. There were two branches of right lower pulmonary venous drainage to the left atrium. There was an exclusion of atrial thrombi.

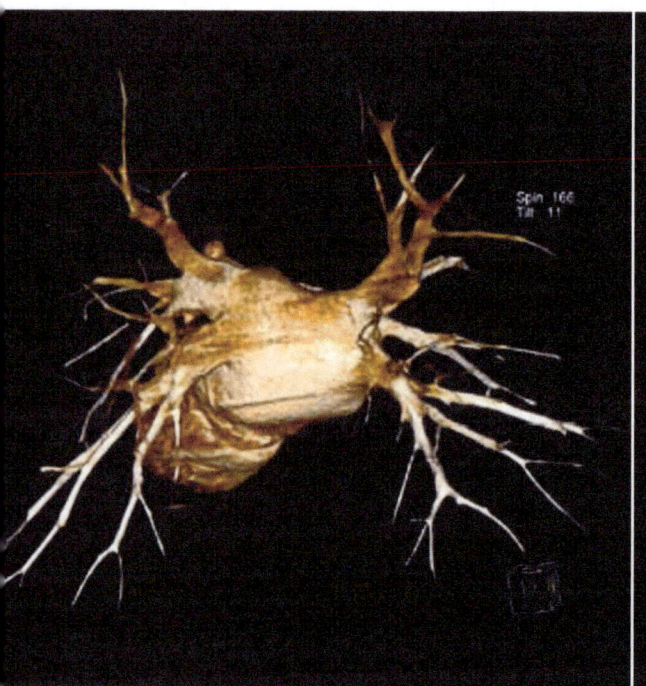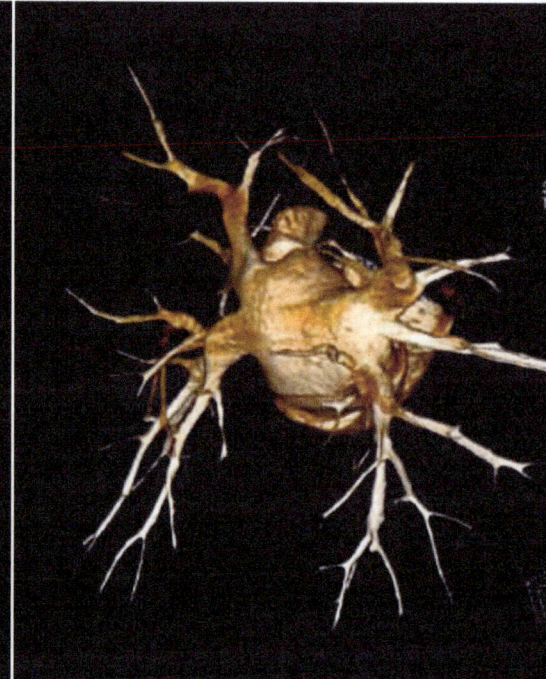

[1] VRT shows the right upper, middle, lower pulmonary venous drainage as well as a branch of right lower pulmonary venous drainage to the left atrium in four-ostium format.

[2] Measurements can be performed by changing angles besides showing pulmonary venous drainage in VRT.

Findings

VRTs revealed separate ostia for upper, middle pulmonary venous on the right side and a branch drainage to the left atrium besides the main right lower pulmonary vein.

VE has verified that the left pulmonary vein had two ostia and the right pulmonary vein had four ostia which was a physiological variation.

Take-home message

Excellent image quality produced by DSCT can exactly demonstrate the anatomy of left atrium and pulmonary veins, provide useful morphological and anatomical information. Furthermore, the technology can be a non-invasive examination of AF and quantitatively analyze the data of patients for RFCA.

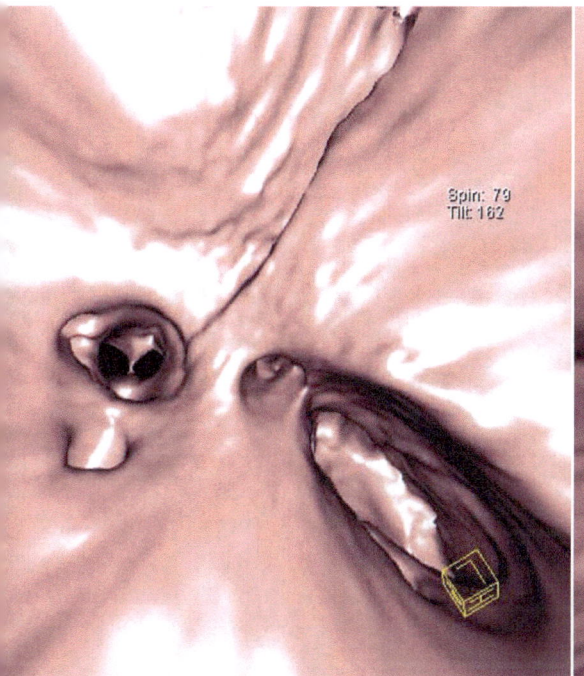 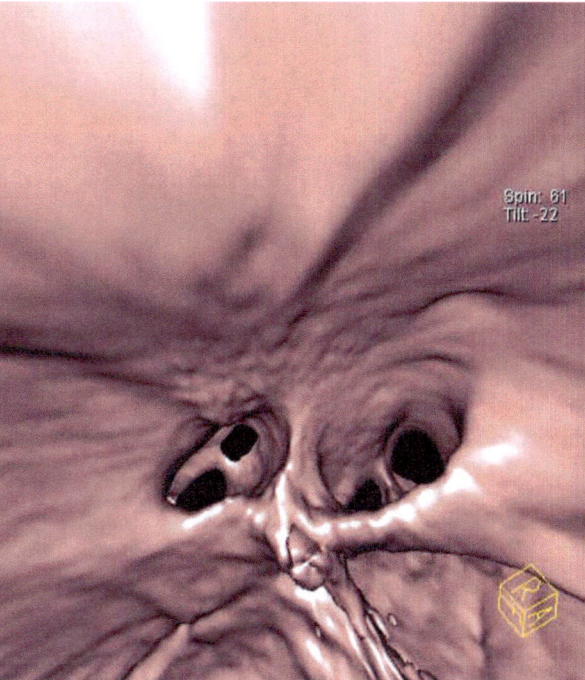

[3] VE shows the right pulmonary venous drainage to the left atrium in four-ostium format.

[4] VE shows the left pulmonary venous drainage to the left atrium in two-ostium format.

Vascular
Aortic Runoff, Abdominal CTA

Foong Koon Cheah
John Huang

Department of Radiology
Singapore General Hospital
Singapore

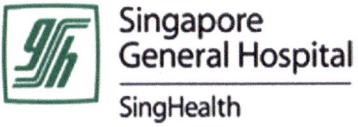
Singapore
General Hospital
SingHealth

Vascular
Aortic Runoff, Abdominal CTA

Basic considerations

Abdominal and peripheral CTA are robust techniques for elective and emergency indications. Examinations require 10 to 15 minutes of room time. Assessment of small peripheral vessels requires a high spatial resolution. We recommend the acquisition of a thin collimated raw dataset. To achieve optimal and reliable contrast enhancement, biphasic injection protocols are preferred as they result in more uniform attenuation, especially if long scan times are needed. The contrast injection time should be about 10% longer than the scan time in order to ensure sufficient contrast enhancement along the entire scan volume. [1]

Scan Parameters

Scan mode	Single Source, non-gated
Scan area	abdomen to symphysis *
Scan direction	cranio-caudal
Scan time	~10 s *
Tube voltage	120 kV
Tube current	190 quality ref. mAs *
Dose modulation	CARE Dose4D
CTDI$_{vol}$	~13 mGy
Rotation time	0.5 s
Pitch	1.2
Slice collimation	0.6 mm
Acquisition	64 x 0.6 mm
Slice width	0.6 mm *
Reconstruction increment	0.3 mm *
Reconstruction kernel	B30f *

* Asian Adaptation by Singapore General Hospital
To assess smaller structures, resolution is improved by the use of a thinner slice thickness.

Tricks

Align the patient's legs and feet close to the isocenter of the scanner and keep the FoV as small as possible. In the case of suspected arterial occlusion, the use of repeated test-bolus scans (instead of bolus tracking) above and below the level of occlusion may help to optimize contrast timing and avoid outrunning the bolus. Automated tube current modulation should be used to minimize radiation. [1]

Pitfalls

High attenuation objects, e.g. calcifications, may mimic stenosis due to blooming artifacts. Window adjustment with window widths up to 1500 HU is most effective to avoid this problem. Editing artifacts like inadvertent vessel removal or inaccurate centerline definition are other relevant pitfalls. These artifacts can be identified with additional views or review of source images. [1]

Contrast Injection Protocol

	Iodine concentration 370 mg I/ml
Injection scheme	Biphasic
Iodine delivery rate	1.85 g/s, 1.48 g/s
CM volume	scan time x 5 ml/s
CM flow rate	5 ml/s, 4 ml/s
Body weight adaptation	no
Bolus timing	bolus tracking **
Bolus tracking threshold	180 HU
ROI position	juxtarenal aorta
Scan delay	7 s
Saline flush volume	60 ml
Saline injection rate	4 ml/s
Needle size	18 G
Injection site	antecubital vein

** Depending on the preference of the individual site, test bolus can be used as an alternative

[1] A.H. Mahnken, J.E. Wildberger, M. Das in [1]

Case 1
Abdominal Aortic Aneurysm

Case history

A 72-year-old male presented with abdominal pain and a pulsatile mass.

Diagnosis/Differential diagnosis

Abdominal aortic aneurysm was detected.

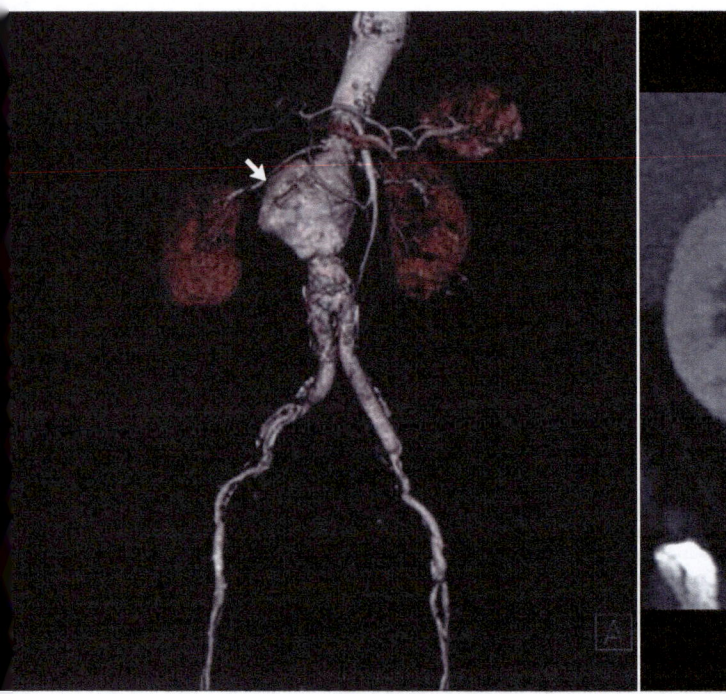

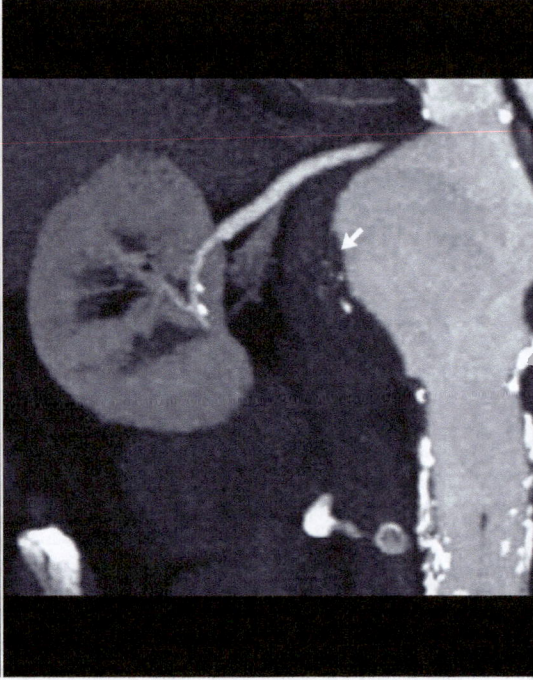

[1] Volume-rendered image shows an infra-renal abdominal aortic aneurysm (arrow).

[2] Coronal maximum intensity projection (MIP) image shows mural thrombus lining the abdominal aortic aneurysm (arrow).

Findings

An infra-renal abdominal aortic aneurysm was found. This was lined by mural thrombus but there was no evidence of contrast extravasation or frank rupture.

Take-home message

DSCT using a single tube allows fast and accurate assessment of the abdominal aorta and branch vessels.

The isotropic dataset obtained can be reformatted in any plane to allow optimum visualization of vascular pathology.

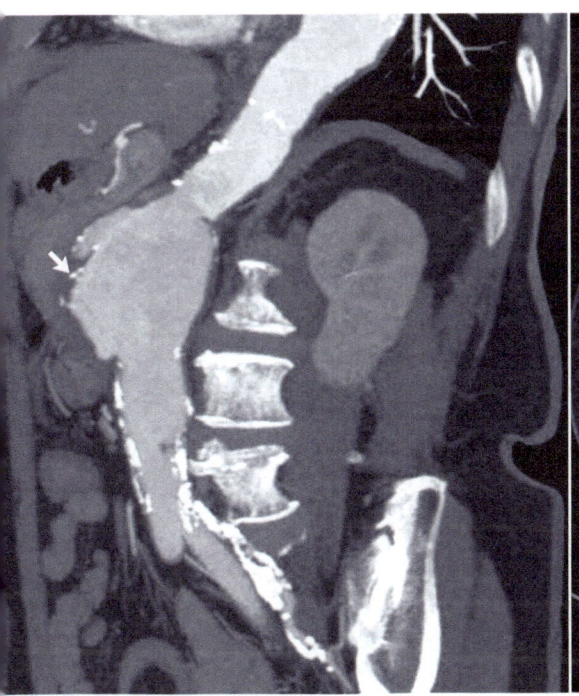 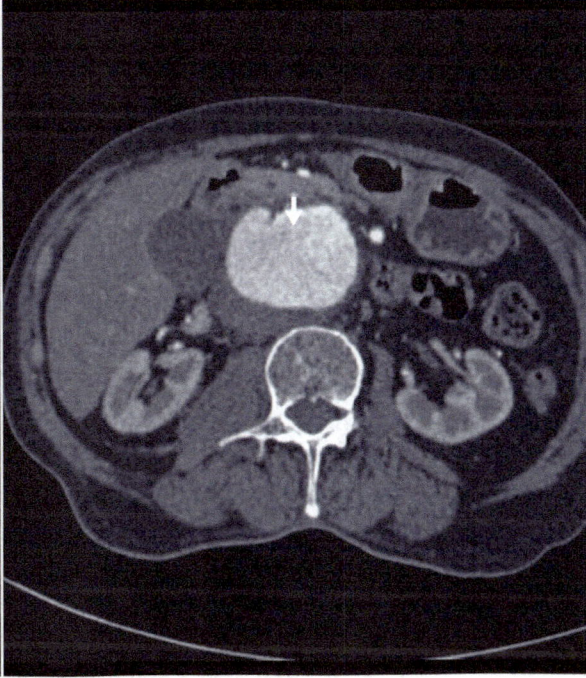

[3] Sagittal MIP image of the abdominal aortic aneurysm (arrow).

[4] Axial source image shows the aneurysm and mural thrombus (arrow).

Case 2
In-stent Restenosis

Case history

A 69-year-old male underwent placement of an aortic stent graft for rupture of an infra-renal abdominal aortic aneurysm. A CT angiogram was performed for follow-up and to detect complications.

Diagnosis / Differential diagnosis

An aortic stent graft in-stent restenosis was detected.

Findings

The stent graft has successfully excluded the aneurysm with no evidence of endoleak. However, mild in-stent restenosis has developed and will require further follow-up.

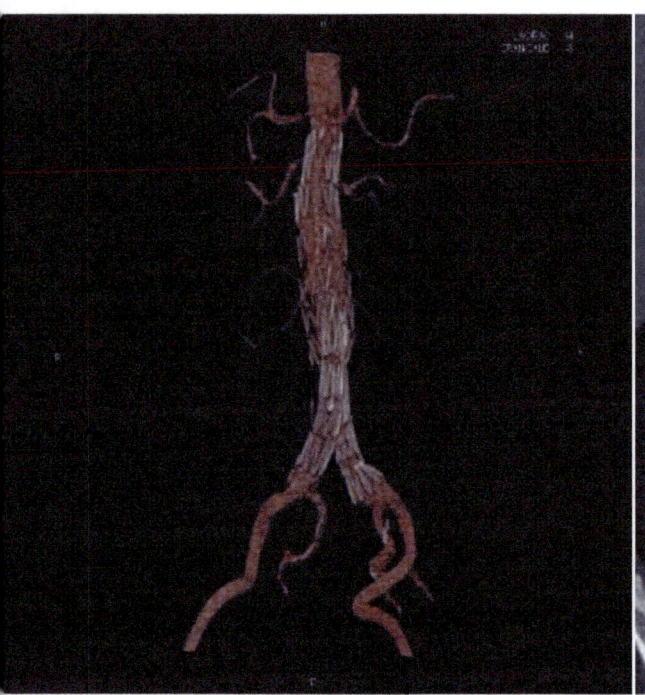

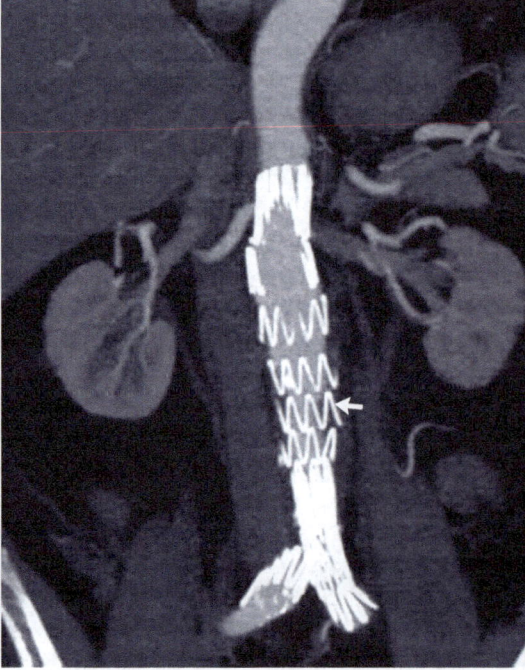

[1] Volume-rendered image of the abdominal aorta showing the stent graft in situ.

[2] Maximum intensity projection (MIP) of the abdominal aorta and stent graft in the coronal plane (arrow).

Take-home message

A monophasic injection should suffice for imaging the abdominal aorta, but if a run-off is required with longer scan times, then a biphasic injection should result in more uniform attenuation.

Follow-up of stent grafts often requires more than one phase. A venous/delayed phase may be useful to detect endoleaks.

Widening of window widths is necessary to avoid blooming artifacts from high-density material such as calcium or metal.

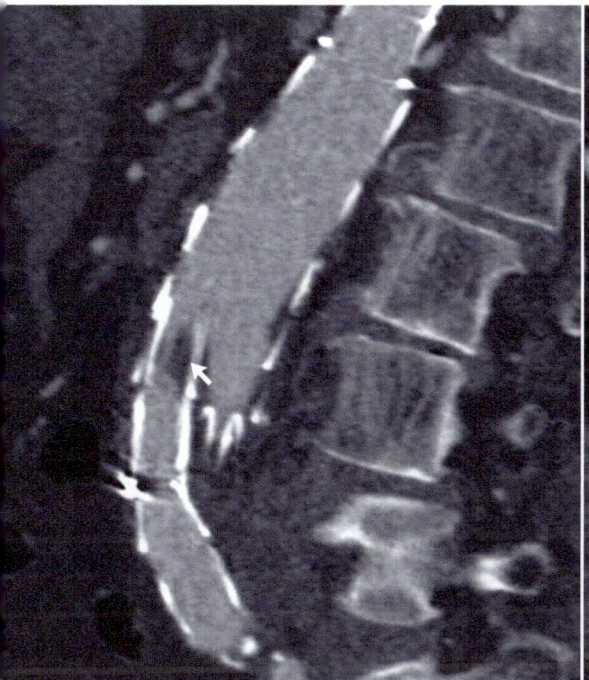
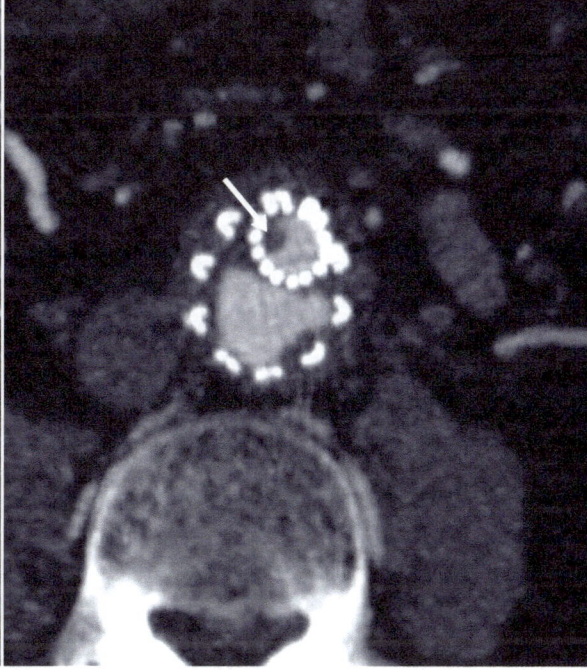

[3] Sagittal multiplanar reformat (MPR) of the bifurcation point of the stent graft showing some mild in-stent restenosis (arrow).

[4] Axial MPR of the stent graft bifurcation point showing mild in-stent restenosis (arrow).

Vascular
Renal CTA

Li Peiling
Chai Ruimei
Wang Qiang
Xu Ke

Department of Radiology
1st Affiliated Hospital of China Medical University
Shenyang, China

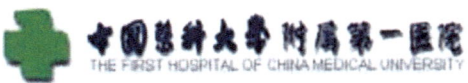

Vascular
Renal CTA

Basic considerations

The protocol is identical to that used on SOMATOM Sensation 64 systems for the evaluation of renal arteries. Due to the variability of the renal artery anatomy, scan coverage area should be at least from the diaphragm to the iliac bifurcation to ensure the inclusion of accessory renal arteries. If renal mass is suspected, consider including non-contrast images and/or a delayed venous-phase scan for the accurate assessment of renal enhancement. Delayed excretory-phase images can also be helpful to evaluate the intrarenal collecting system, ureters, and bladder. [1]

Scan Parameters

Scan mode	Single Source, non-gated
Scan area	diaphragm to iliac bifurcation
Scan direction	cranio-caudal
Scan time	~14 s*
Tube voltage	120 kV
Tube current	250 quality ref. mAs*
Dose modulation	CARE Dose4D
$CTDI_{vo}$	~20 mGy*
Rotation time	0.5 s
Pitch	1.2*
Slice collimation	0.6 mm
Acquisition	64 x 0.6 mm
Slice width	1.0 mm*
Reconstruction increment	0.5 mm*
Reconstruction kernel	B30f*

* **Asian Adaptation by**
1st Affiliated Hospital of China Medical University
Since the patient population in Asia is typically slimmer that in the US and Europe, faster pitch value can be used without reaching the system limits.

Tricks

Reconstruct a smaller FoV just focusing on the kidneys with overlapping reconstructions. Coronal and sagittal multi-planar reformats and 3D reconstructions can provide additional information and are particularly helpful for communicating findings to referring physicians. Use of a smoother kernel (e.g. B20) can further improve quality of 3D reconstruction. [1]

Pitfalls

Test bolus method should not be used to avoid opacification of renal parenchyma prior to CT angiogram. To avoid images that are too noisy, consider increasing the quality ref. mAs in obese patients. [1]

Contrast Injection Protocol

	Iodine concentration 370 mg I/ml
Injection scheme	Monophasic
Iodine delivery rate	1.5 g/s
CM volume	80 ml
CM flow rate	4.1 ml/s
Body weight adaptation	no
Bolus timing	bolus tracking
Bolus tracking threshold	150 HU
ROI position	aorta, 2 cm above diaphragm
Scan delay	4 s
Saline flush volume	60 ml
Saline injection rate	4.1 ml/s
Needle size	18 G
Injection site	antecubital vein

[1] R. Hartman, T.J. Vrtiska, C. McCollough in [1]

Case 1
Hypertension Disease

Case history

A 41-year-old female presented with a hypertension for 3 years and was insensitive to antihypertensive drugs. A renal hypertension was suspected by the clinician.

Diagnosis / Differential diagnosis

The renal CT angiography (CTA) indicated that the bilateral renal arteries were both normal.

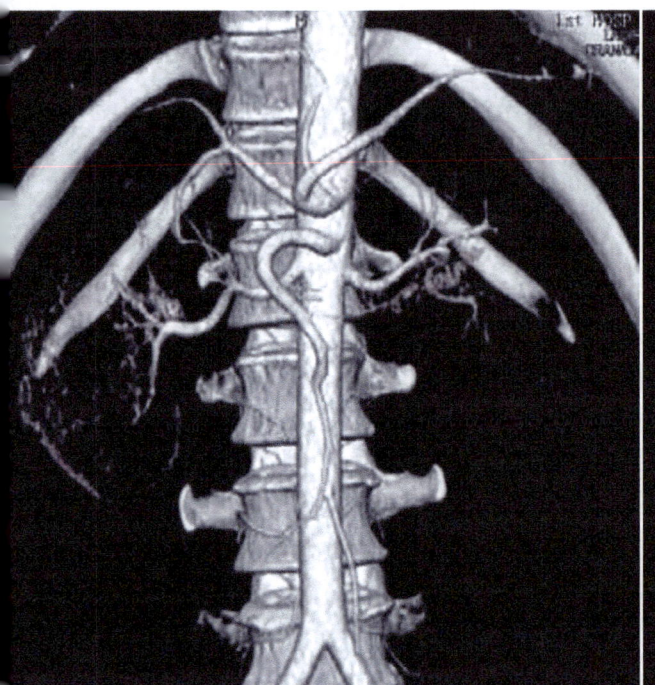

[1] CTA image of kidney prior to bone subtraction.

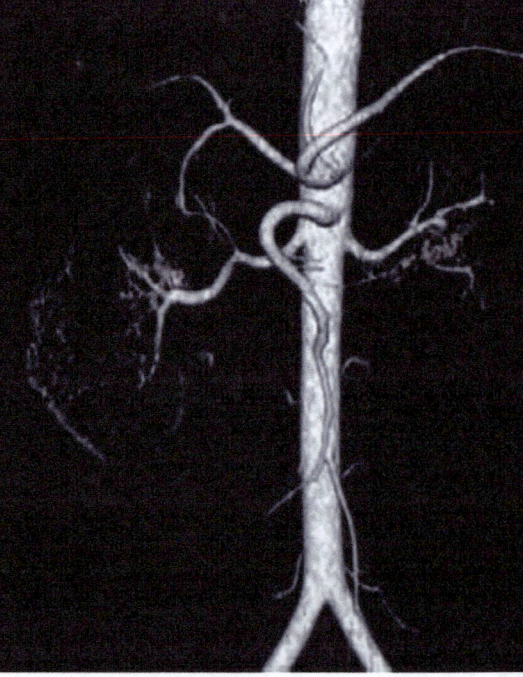

[2] CTA image of kidney with automatic bone subtraction technique.

Findings

The bilateral renal arteries had a normal morphology and the respective lumens were unobstructed. No stenosis or dilation were seen.

Take-home message

CT acquisition and postprocessing allows automatic removal of bone to facilitate the visualization of the vascular anatomy.

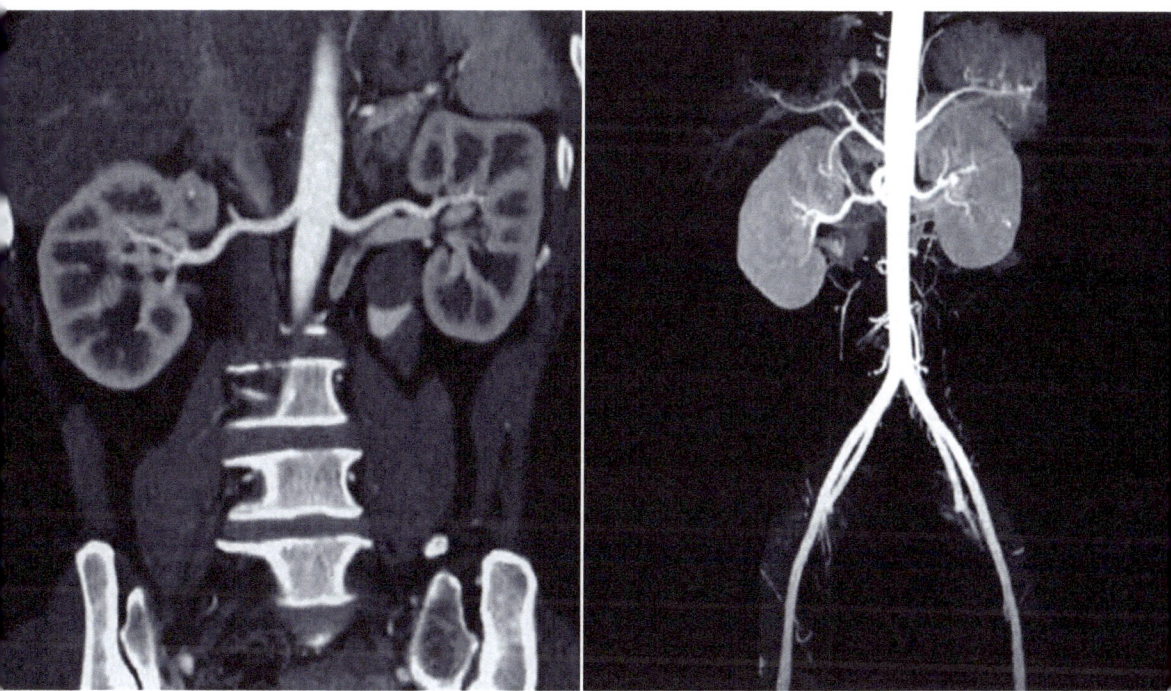

[3] Curved image of bilateral renal arteries.

[4] MIP image of renal artery.

Case 2
Trauma

Case history

A 45-year-old male presented with a lumbar trauma and hematuria.

Diagnosis / Differential diagnosis

The bilateral renal arteries were both normal.

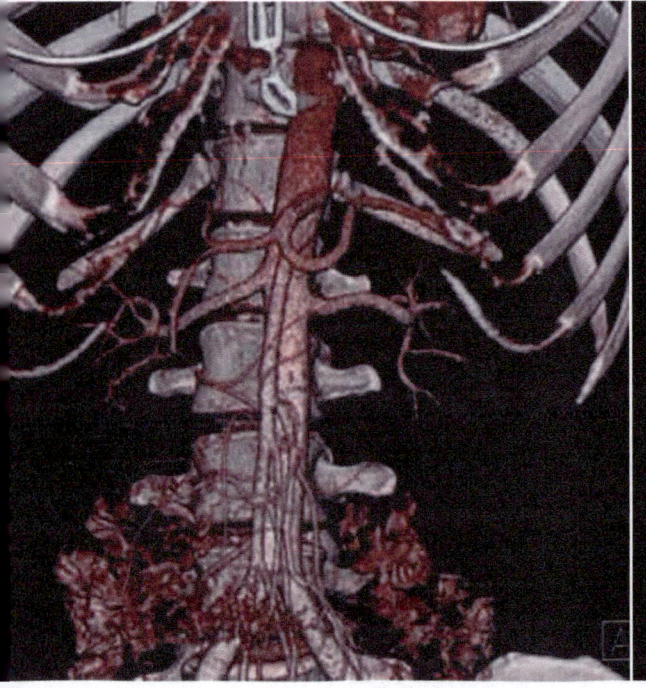 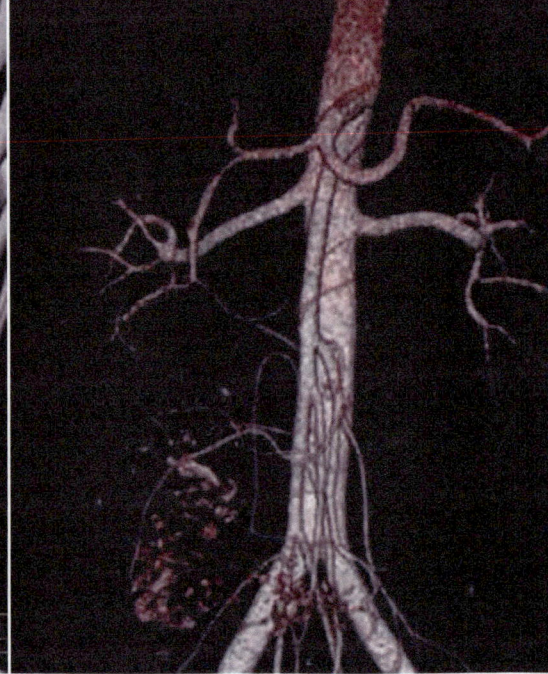

[1] CTA image of kidney prior to bone subtraction.

[2] CTA image of kidney with automatic bone subtraction technique.

Findings

The bilateral renal arteries had a normal morphology and the respective lumens were unobstructed. No stenosis or dilatation was seen.

Take-home message

CT acquisition and postprocessing allows automatic removal of bone and calcified plaque to facilitate the visualization of the vascular anatomy.

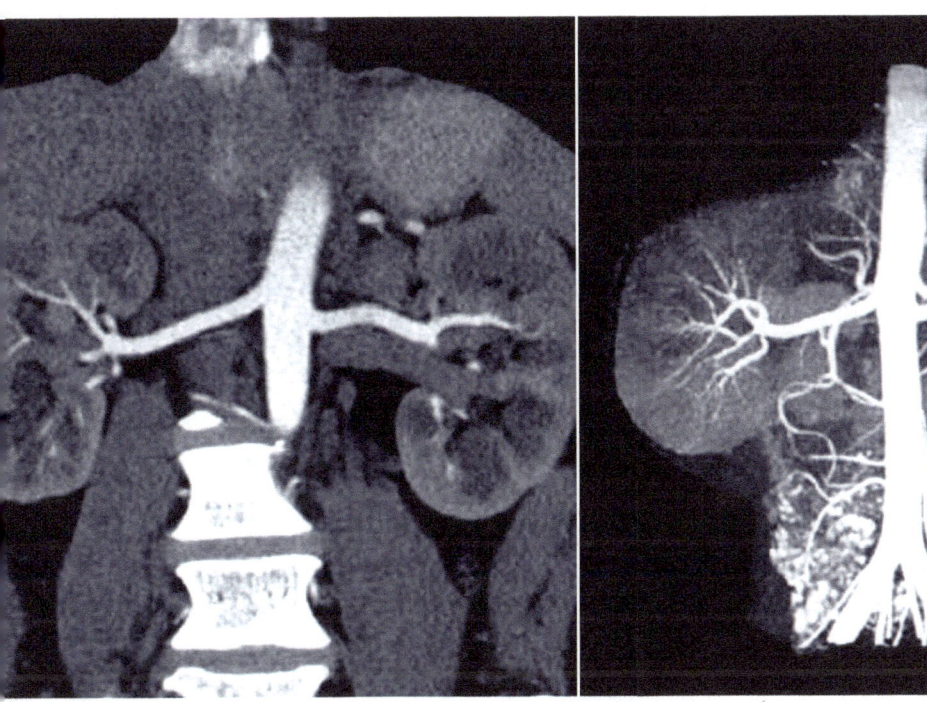

[3] Curved image of bilateral renal arteries.

[4] MIP image of renal artery.

Vascular
Peripheral Runoff

Cheong-Il Shin
Eun-Ah Park
Whal Lee

Department of Radiology
Seoul National University Hospital
Seoul, Korea

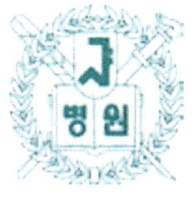

Vascular
Peripheral Runoff

Basic considerations

There is a wide variation in contrast material bolus transit speed ranging from 2.9–17.7 cm/sec, especially in patients with peripheral arterial occlusive disease. Because it is virtually impossible to accurately predict the contrast material transit time for any individual patient, test bolus method using 2 separate mini-boluses would be ideal not to fail the exam. However, bolus tracking method is a more reasonable approach in a busy situation because it is so easy and simple that a lot of exams can be handled in limited time. Regarding the scan parameters, lowest table speed of 3 cm/sec is mandatory to overcome the outrun. Considering that the Asian population is relatively short with average scan length 120 cm, scan time is estimated to about 40 seconds.

Scan Parameters

Scan mode	Single Source, non-gated
Scan area	renal artery to feet
Scan direction	cranio-caudal
Scan time	~40 s
Tube voltage	100 kV
Tube current	160 quality ref. mAs
Dose modulation	CARE Dose 4D
$CTDI_{vol}$	~6 mGy
Rotation time	0.5 s
Pitch	0.8
Slice collimation	0.6 mm
Acquisition	64 x 0.6 mm
Slice width	1.5 mm / 3 mm
Reconstruction increment	1 mm / 3 mm
Reconstruction kernel	B25f / B30f

Asian Adaptation by Seoul National University Hospital
Due to the slimmer population in Asia, typically lower kV values at an adjusted quality ref. mAs level are used which leads to lower $CTDI_{vol}$ values.

Tricks

Even in the protocol of fast acquisition, make sure not to reduce total volume of contrast materials. In the protocol of fast acquisition, it is better to set the longer scan delay time instead of reducing total volume of contrast materials in order to keep maximal enhancement of lower extremity arteries. Another consideration for achieving high arterial enhancement is using a low kVp.

Pitfalls

Be aware that even with table speed < 3 cm/s, it is possible to outrun the bolus. Therefore, an additional preprogrammed subsequent acquisition immediately after the first scan is recommended – from the knees to the feet, but only if the technologist does not see adequate opacification of pedal vessels.

Contrast Injection Protocol

	Iodine concentration 370 mg I/ml
Injection scheme	Monophasic
Iodine delivery rate	1.48 g/s
CM volume	120 ml
CM flow rate	4 ml/s
Body weight adaptation	no
Bolus timing	n.a.
Bolus tracking threshold	150 HU
ROI position	abdominal aorta
Scan delay	8 s
Saline flush volume	70 ml
Saline injection rate	4 ml/s
Needle size	18 G
Injection site	antecubital vein

Case 1
Acute Peripheral Arterial Occlusion

Case history

A 65-year-old male with underlying melanoma presented with a tingling sensation in the left leg as well as coldness for one month, just after beginning chemotherapy.

Diagnosis / Differential diagnosis

Given his clinical history, acute peripheral arterial occlusion was suspected. In this particular patient, differential diagnosis would include acute embolic occlusion and acute arterial thrombosis induced by chemotherapy.

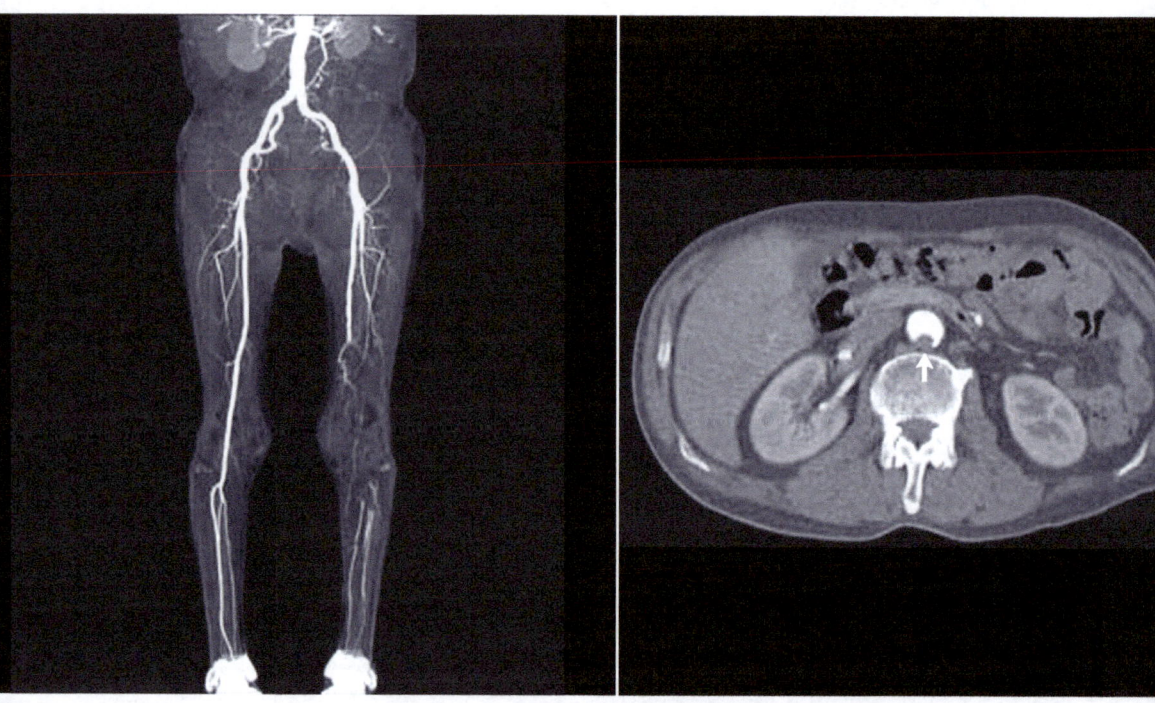

[1] MIP image after bone removal. Note the total occlusion from the distal femoral artery to the proximal calf arteries in the left leg.

[2] Axial source image at the level of infrarenal aorta. Small thrombus is attached to the posterior wall of the aorta (arrow). However, this is not seen on the reconstructed image.

Findings

Total occlusion of the left distal superficial femoral to the popliteal artery as well as tibio-fibular trifurcation was noted. At the infrarenal aorta, newly developed thrombus was identified. Thus, the presumptive diagnosis was embolic occlusion with embolic source from the chemotherapy-induced thrombi on the aorta. The appearance of the arteries elsewhere was almost normal with minimal plaque burden.

Take-home message

MIP image provides the best visualization of the highest attenuated structures, as in enhancing vascular structures, which allows for quick and accurate diagnosis of lower extremity CT angiography. However, we must keep in mind that MIP display can also obscure eccentric lesions.

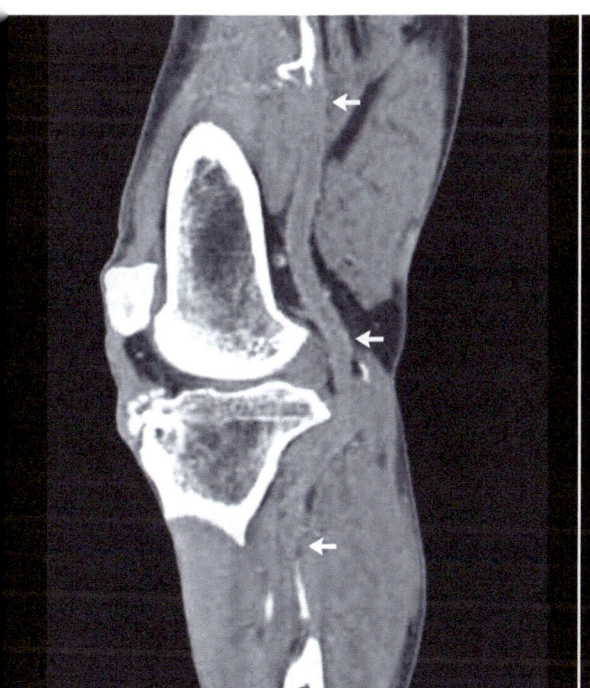

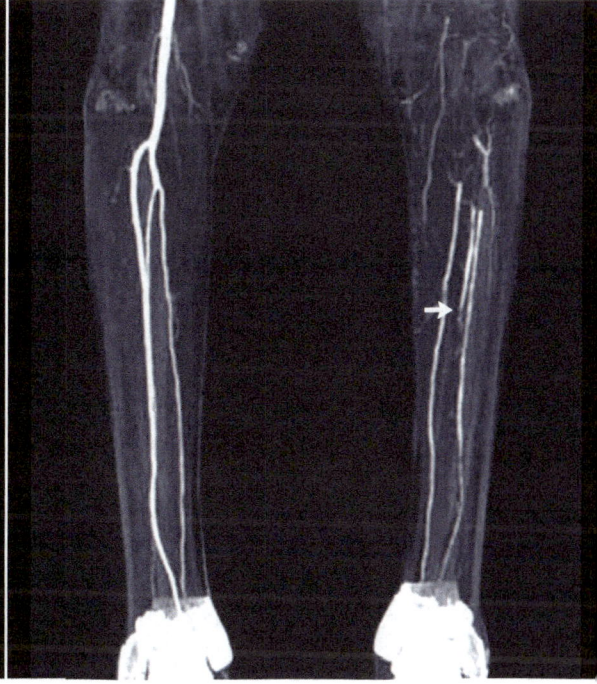

[3] Curved MPR image of the occluded segment. Long segmental intraluminal filling defect is well demonstrated (arrows).

[4] MIP image of lower legs. Another distal embolic occlusion is noted in the left peritoneal artery (arrow).

Case 2
Young Male with Leg Claudication

Case history

A 26-year-old male presented with bilateral leg claudication for 3 years. He was a 20-pack-year smoker. He denied trauma history and underlying disease.

Diagnosis/Differential diagnosis

The diagnosis was not conclusive. However, there was a high possibility of thromboangiitis obliterans involving bilateral iliofemoral arteries. Vasculitis from unknown cause could also be included in the differential diagnosis.

Findings

Bilateral proximal to mid superficial femoral arteries were segmentally occluded and reconstituted via fine collaterals which were symmetric. Bilateral proximal external iliac arteries also showed focal severe stenosis. No calcified plaques were shown. Distal runoff was patent. There were no abnormal findings in the abdominal aorta and splanchnic vessels.

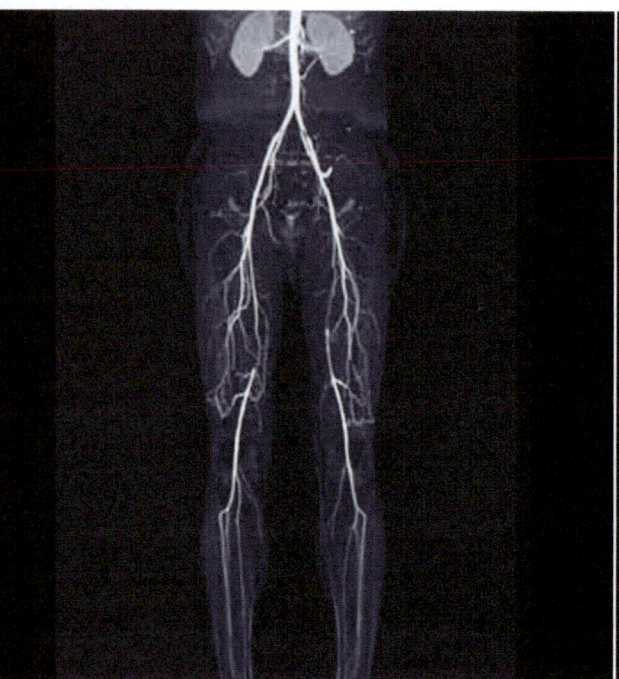 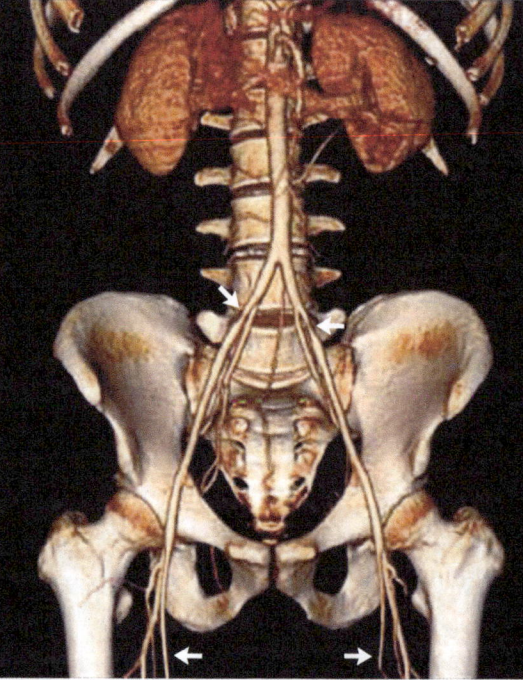

[1] MIP image after bone removal. MIP image provides excellent overview of the lower extremity arterial system serving as a map of disease extent.

[2] VR image of the aortoiliac artery. Focal concentric stenosis of both external iliac arteries are well visualized (upper arrows). Also, both proximal superficial arteries are diffusely narrowed (lower arrows).

Take-home message

Visualization of vessel wall status, along with the simultaneous evaluation of adjacent structures and its anatomic relationships is an absolute benefit of CT angiography, which cannot be provided by conventional angiography. Thromboangiitis obliterans is a non-atherosclerotic segmental inflammatory vascular disease that most commonly affects small- and medium-sized vessels of the arms and legs with male predominance. However, it rarely involves the iliac artery in addition to the occlusive lesion in the leg arteries with an incidence of only 6.5%. The obliterative lesion of the iliac artery might owe its cause to a direct proximal progression of thromboangiitic obliterans of the femoral artery or to skip progression. Our patient initially presented with bilateral occlusion of the femoral artery without involvement of the iliac artery 2 years ago (image not provided) and showed skip progression of bilateral iliac arteries.

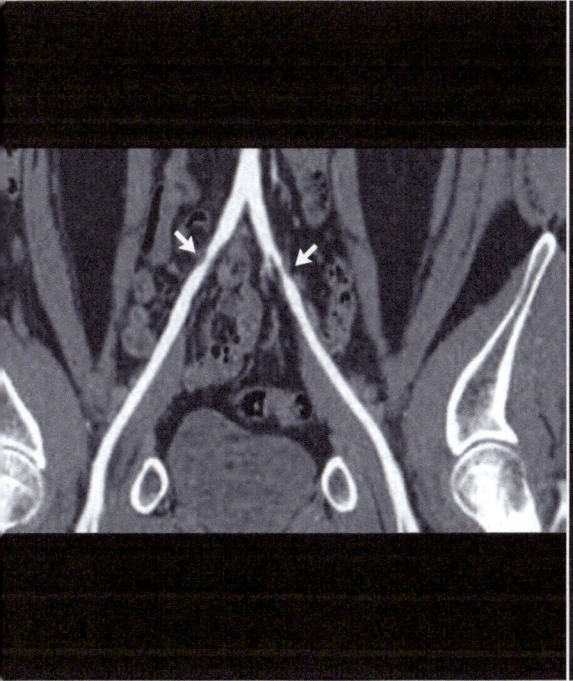

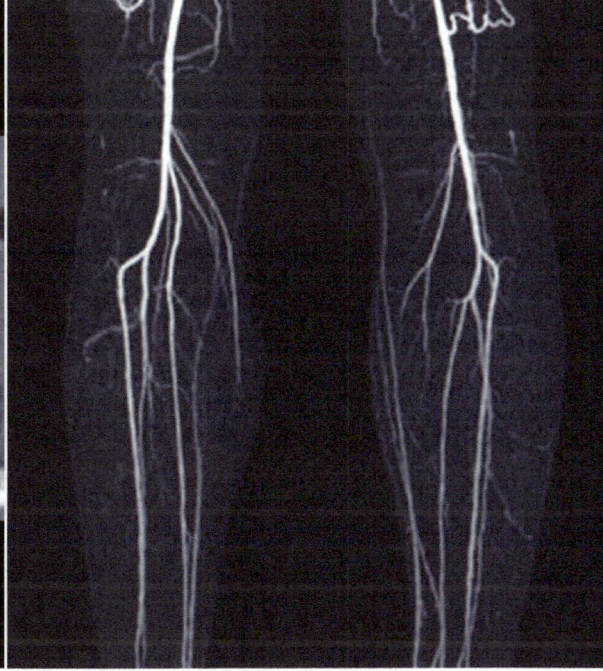

[3] Curved MPR image can provide information of extraluminal abnormality. No plaques nor vessel wall thickening were noted in both external iliac artery segments.

[4] MIP image of upper and lower legs. Both femoral arteries show segmental occlusion. Distal runoff is good. Minimal venous contamination in the greater saphenous veins is noted.

Vascular
Brain Perfusion

Seungbae Hwang
Gongyong Jin
Hyosung Kwak

Department of Radiology,
Chonbuk National University Hospital
Jeonju, Republic of Korea

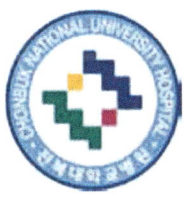

Vascular
Brain Perfusion

Basic considerations

PBV imaging is based on a subtraction of NECT and CTA data. Therefore, the same field of view and identical reconstruction parameters are required for both examinations. Although the software can correct to some extent for patient movement between the two scans, movement of the head should be strictly avoided. To calculate the PBV, a CTA scan with sufficient parenchymal and venous enhancement is required. Therefore the cerebral transit time (5 – 6 s) has to be added to the CM arrival time in the cerebral arteries if a test-bolus technique is used to determine the scan delay. [1]

Scan Parameters	PBV	Perfusion CT
Scan mode	Single Source, non-gated	DynMulti, Single Source, non-gated
Scan area	aortic arch to superior sagittal sinus	brain
Scan direction	caudo-cranial	caudo-cranial
Scan time	10 s	40 s
Tube voltage	120 kV	80 kV
Tube current	130 eff. mAs	270 eff. mAs
Dose modulation	no	no
$CTDI_{vol}$	~ 20 mGy	~430 mGy
Rotation time	0.5 s	1.0 s
Pitch	0.8	n.a.
Slice collimation	0.6 mm	20.8 mm
Acquisition	64 x 0.6 mm	24 x 1.2 mm
Slice width	1 mm	10 mm
Reconstruction increment	0.7 mm	1.0 mm
Reconstruction kernel	H22f	H30s

Asian Adaptation by Chonbuk National University Hospital

Tricks

If a perfusion CT is required, it should be done before the cerebral CTA. The scan delay for the CTA can also be determined from the dynamic perfusion scan. Select the time to peak enhancement in the superior sagittal sinus as scan delay. In this case, no additional delay time is required to account for cerebral transit time. [1]

Pitfalls

Do not forget to add the start delay of the PCT scan when determining the CTA delay from an arterial vessel in the PCT scan. If the CTA scan that is to be used to calculate the PBV is started too early, it results in overestimation of the infarction. [1]

Contrast Injection Protocol	PBV	Perfusion CT
Iodine concentration 370 mg I/ml		
Injection scheme	Monophasic	Monophasic
Iodine delivery rate	1.48 g/s	2.59 g/s
CM volume	80 ml	50 ml
CM flow rate	4 ml/s	7 ml/s
Body weight adaptation	no	no
Bolus timing	test bolus **	–
Bolus tracking threshold	n.a.	–
ROI position	basilar artery	basilar artery
Scan delay	peak time plus 6 s	5 s
Saline flush volume	60 ml	50 ml
Saline injection rate	4 ml/s	7 ml/s
Needle size	18 G	18 G
Injection site	antecubital vein	antecubital vein

[1] H. Seifarth, T. Fischer, R. Fischbach, S. Kloska in [1]

Case 1 (PBV)
Cerebral Infarction

Case history

73-year-old woman presented with slurred speech; onset was one day prior to examination. On physical examination she presented with right-sided hemiparesis.

Diagnosis / Differential diagnosis

We diganosed an acute left middle cerebral infarction.

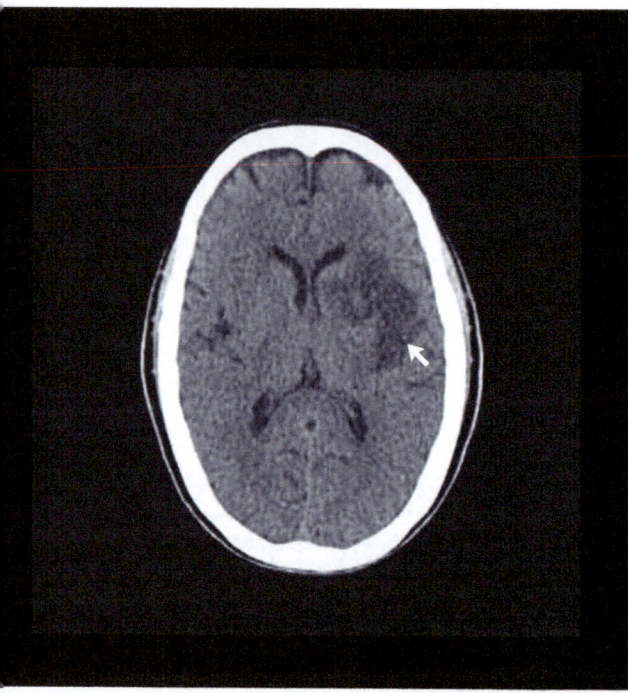
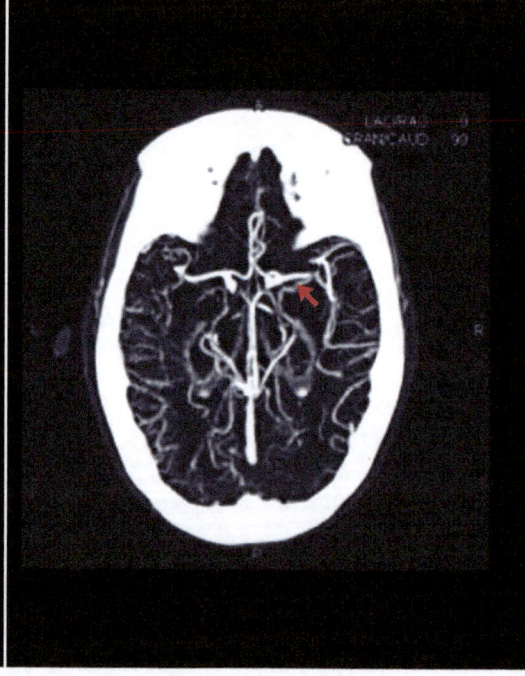

[1] Pre-contrast brain CT shows ill-defined hypodense lesion (arrow) in left basal ganglia.

[2] MIP of a CTA shows severe stenosis at middle cerebral artery.

Findings

Pre-enhanced brain CT showed ill-defined hypodense lesion in left basal ganglia. CTA showed a stenosis of left middle cerebral artery and normal carotid artery. The PBV image showed a large perfusion deficit in the left basal ganglia.

Take-home message

Because of the coverage of the entire brain and the upper aortic arch, perfusion deficit at brain parenchyma and absence or presence of carotid artery stenosis can be detected simultaneously using brain CTA.

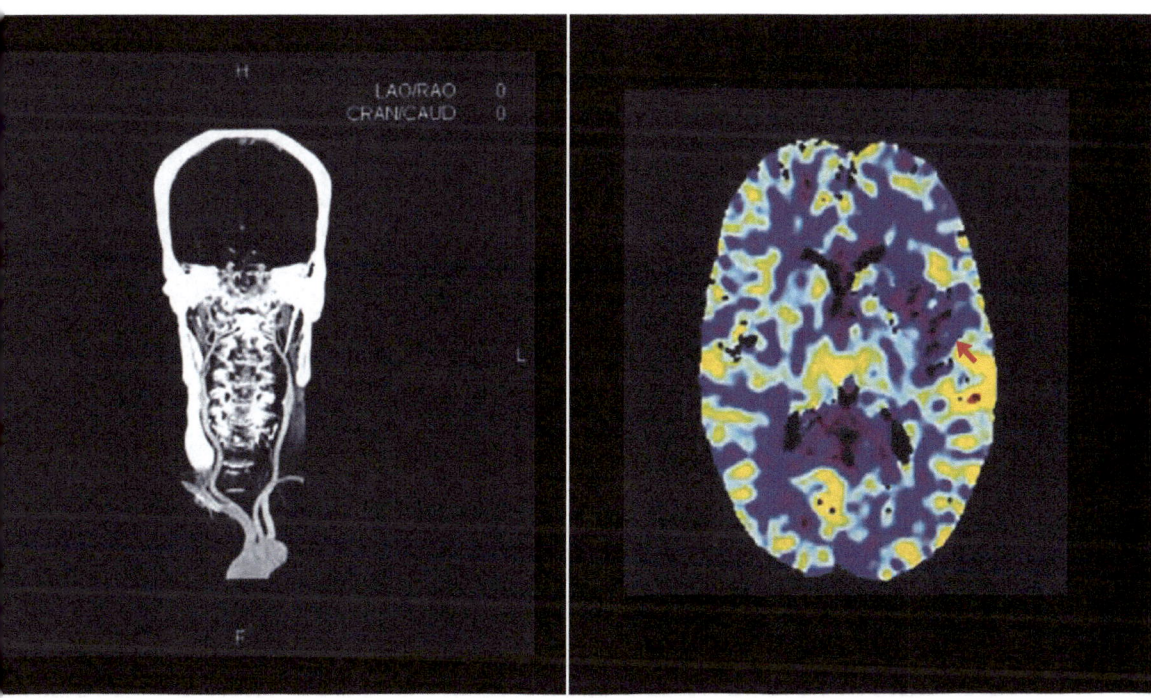

[3] Coronal MIP shows normal carotid artery.

[4] Large extent of the perfusion deficit can be seen on the PBV data.

Case 2 Perfusion CT
Ischemic Infarction

Case history

A 57-year-old male presented with blurred vision; the onset had been 2 months previously.

Diagnosis/Differential diagnosis

We diagnosed subacute cerebral infarction in right posterior MCA territory and chronic infarction in left posterior MCA territory.

Findings

Pre-enhanced brain CT showed ill-defined hypodense lesions in both posterior MCA territories. On post-contrast MR imaging, parenchymal enhancement with gyral pattern in right posterior MCA territory demonstrated subacute infarction, and cystic encephalomalacic change in left posterior MCA territory demonstrated chronic

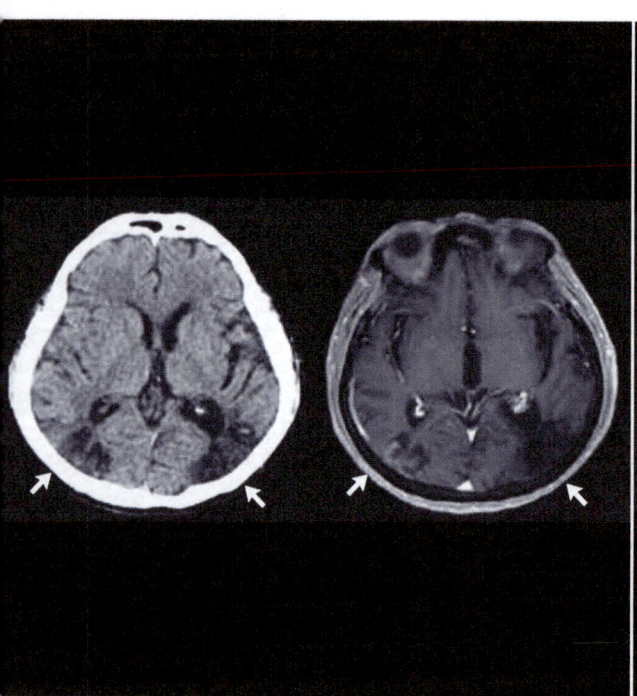 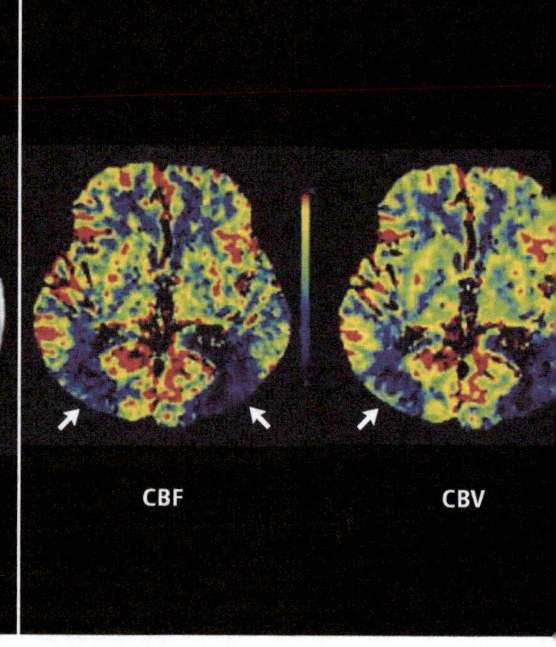

[1] Pre-contrast brain CT (left) showed ill-defined hypodense lesion (arrows) in both posterior MCA territory. Post-contrast-enhanced MR imaging (right) showed parenchymal enhancement with gyral pattern in right side and cystic encephalomalacic change in left side.

[2] The perfusion deficit (arrows) can be seen in both posterior MCA territory on CBF (Cerebral Blood Flow) and CBV (Cerebral Blood Volume) map.

infarction. The perfusion CT with CBF and CBV map showed a perfusion deficit in infarcted areas. MR angiography showed nearly complete occlusion of the left middle cerebral artery. TTP map showed delayed perfusion in the left MCA territory, except for perfusion defect in infarcted areas.

Take-home message

CBV and CBF depicts the perfusion deficit correlating to the TTP in axial slice in the acute and subacute phase of an ischemic infarction. TTP in an ischemic infarction showed a delayed perfusion compared to normal TTP.

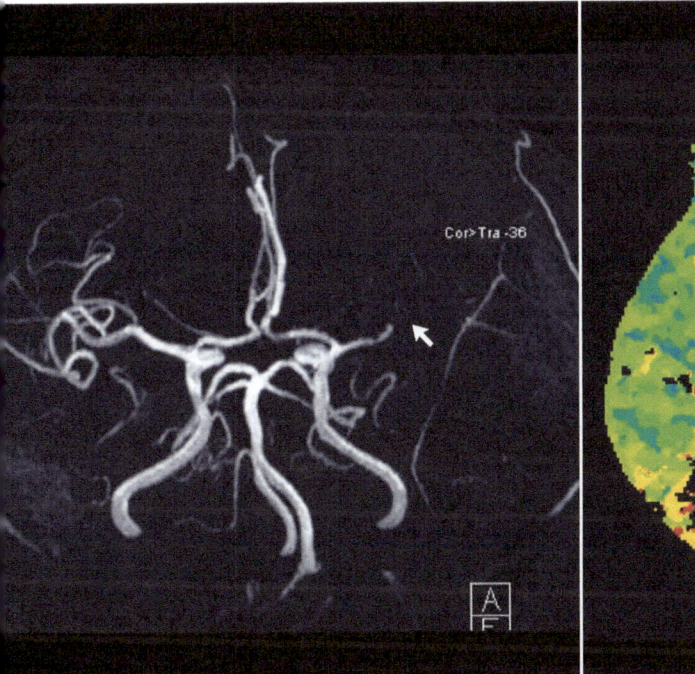

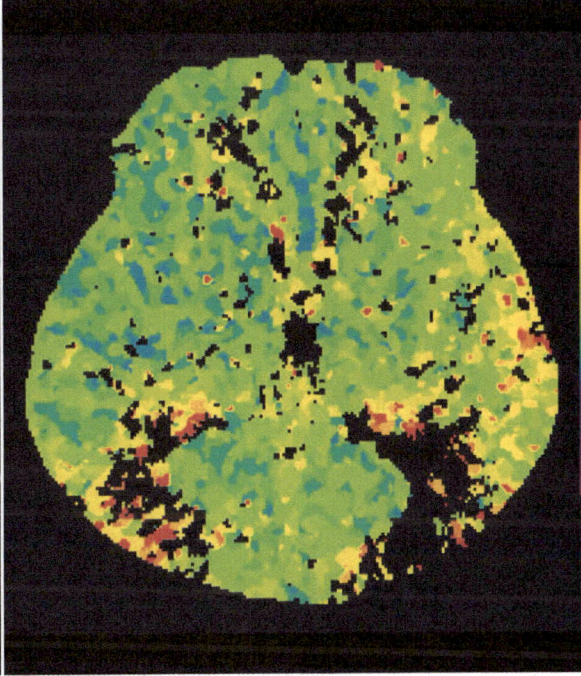

[3] MR angiography showed nearly complete occlusion of left middle cerebral artery (arrow).

[4] TTP map showed delayed perfusion in the whole left middle cerebral artery territory, especially marked perfusion delay in infarcted area.

Dual Energy CT Applications

Dual Energy
CTA of Head and Neck

Feng Yun
Liu Ming
Xue Jianping
Li Yuhua

Department of Radiology
Xinhua Hospital
Shanghai, China

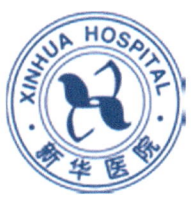

Dual Energy
CTA of Head and Neck

Basic considerations

Good image quality always depends on good pre-scan preparations: A comfortable headrest position for compliant and an effective fixation of non-compliant patients is mandatory to avoid motion artifacts, even at a high pitch and 0.33 s gantry rotation time. Dental implants tend to cause severe beam hardening artifacts. Individual head positioning with the adjustable head-rest can avoid artifacts over the carotid bulb, one of the regions with the highest clinical relevance.

Depending on the indication, good enhancement of arteries (only) or arteries and veins has to be achieved. Start delay has to be adjusted depending on desired contrast-phase. [1]

Scan Parameters

Scan mode	Spiral Dual Energy with Dual Source
Scan area	all supra-aortic vessels or intracranial
Scan direction	caudo-cranial
Scan time	~10 s*
Tube voltage A/B	140 kV / 80 kV
Tube current A/B	55 quality ref. mAs / 234 quality ref. mAs
Dose modulation	CARE Dose 4D
$CTDI_{vol}$	~7 mGy*
Rotation time	0.33 s
Pitch	0.7
Slice collimation	0.6 mm
Acquisition	64 x 0.6 mm
Slice width	1 mm*
Reconstruction increment	0.5 mm*
Reconstruction kernel	D30f*

* **Asian Adaptation by Shanghai Xinhua Hospital**
Compared to dose values seen in the US and Europe, $CTDI_{vol}$ dose values in Asia are lower.

Tricks

Timing of contrast agent injection can be adjusted to achieve pure arterial enhancement to evaluate arteries with less venous overlay. To get the best enhancement to evaluate all intracranial vasculature, delay can be set between 30 and 35 seconds (e.g. to rule out venous thrombosis). Dual topograms in anterior-posterior and lateral projection help positioning. [1]

Pitfalls

Missing contrast bolus by placing monitoring ROI outside the aorta. Using cranio-caudal scan direction for early arterial phase scanning (long range table movement may waste valuable seconds). Removed calcified plaque may result in irregularities of the vessel wall mimicking a more complex aneurysm architecture with lobulations and "baby-aneurysm". [1]

Contrast Injection Protocol

	Iodine concentration 370 mg I/ml
Injection scheme	Monophasic
Iodine delivery rate	2.2 g/s
CM volume	80 ml
CM flow rate	6 ml/s
Body weight adaptation	yes
Bolus timing	bolus tracking **
Bolus tracking threshold	200 HU
ROI position	ascending aorta
Scan delay	4 s for pure arterial 25 s for arteries and venous
Saline flush volume	100 ml
Saline injection rate	6 ml/s
Needle size	18 G
Injection site	antecubital vein

** Depending on the preference of the individual site, test bolus can be used as an alternative

[1] D. Morhard, T. Johnson, C.R. Becker in [1]

Case 1
Multi-segmental Stenosis: Cervical Vessels

Case history

A 67-year-old male presented with aphasia
for three days. A non-contrast CT scan showed
multiple lacunar infarctions in the bilateral basal
ganglion area and brain stem.

Diagnosis / Differential diagnosis

Mild segmental stenosis of the right carotid
bifurcation and bilateral middle cerebral arteries
due to arteriosclerosis were shown. Multiple
calcified plaques were found at intra- and extra-
cranial vessels with or without luminal stenosis.

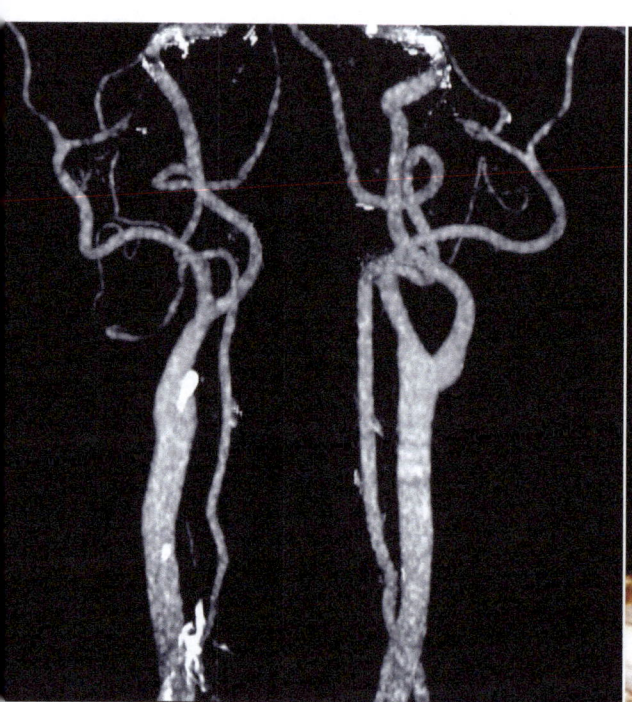
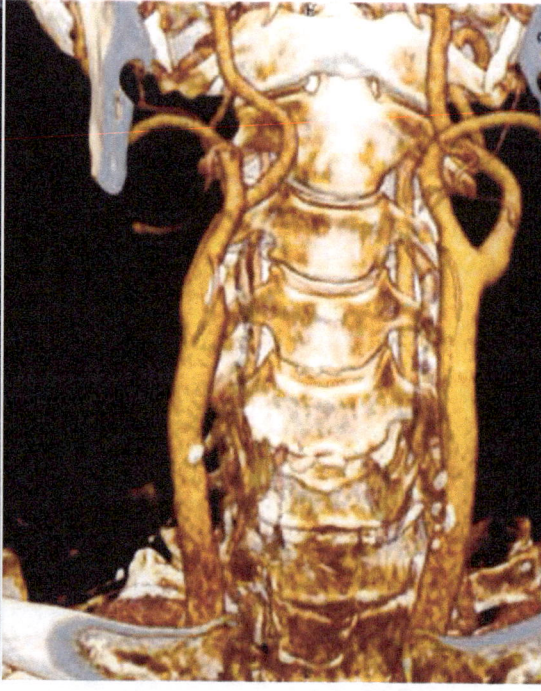

[1] MIP reconstruction after bone removal shows a hard
calcified plaque at the bifurcation of the right common carotid
artery.

[2] VR image without the bone removal shows a plaque at the
bifurcation of the right CCA.

Findings

Multiple calcified plaques were found at the right bifurcation and the left proximal common carotid arteries, the plaque also visualized at intracranial vessels. Mild stenosis at the segments of the arteries due to the plaque appeared quite clearly based on the bone-removal reconstruction.

Take-home message

The bone-removal reconstruction with the DE technique can remove most of calcified plaque on the lumen of the artery. Sometimes both of the processed and unprocessed bone images should be evaluated carefully to confirm the size and the extent of the plaque. This technique plays an important role in the evaluation of stenoses or aneurysms of the intracranial Willis circle.

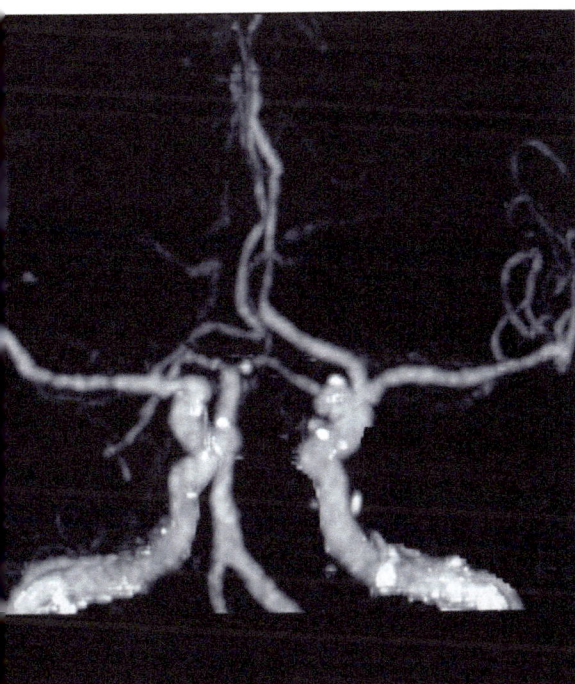

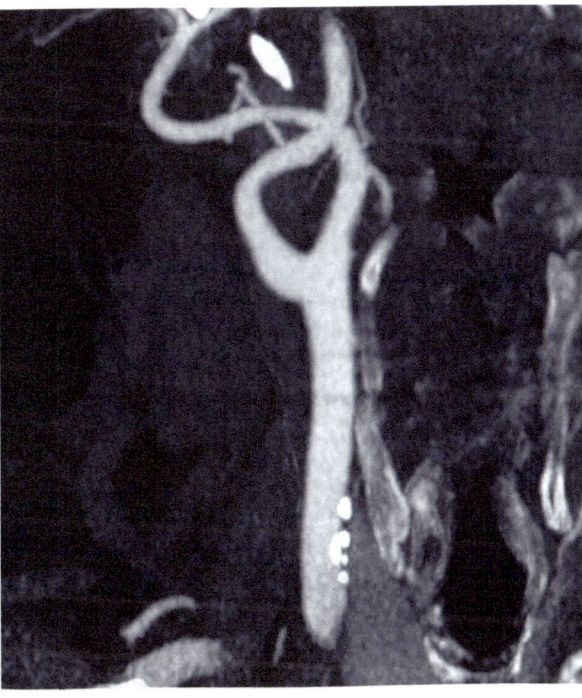

[3] Bone-removed VR image shows multiple calcified plaque and mild stenosis at the bilateral carotid and the middle cerebral arteries.

[4] Oblique thick MIP reconstruction image demonstrates the multiple calcified plaque at the proximal CCA.

Case 2
Multi-segmental Stenosis: Intracranial Vessels

Case history

A 73-year-old female presented with aphasia and hemiplegia on the right side of her body for four days. Magnetic resonance imaging revealed multiple lacunar infarct lesions in the bilateral basal ganglia.

Diagnosis/Differential diagnosis

The common carotid arteries (CCA) and the carotid bifurcation were normal on both sides with no evidence of stenosis or occlusion. The CT angiography showed a significant stenosis at the segment of the right internal carotid of the Willis circle and mild multi-segmental stenosis of the middle cerebral artery.

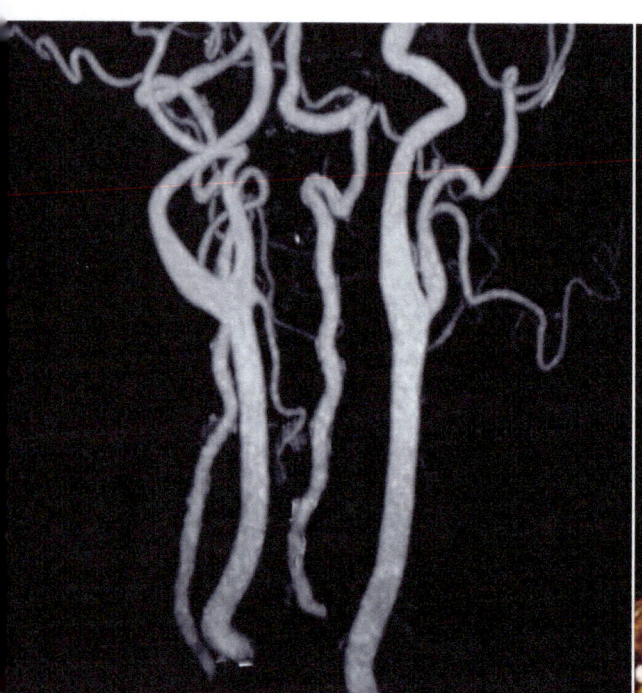

[1] Dual Energy bone removal MIP image demonstrates the intra- and extra-cranial vascular without bone.

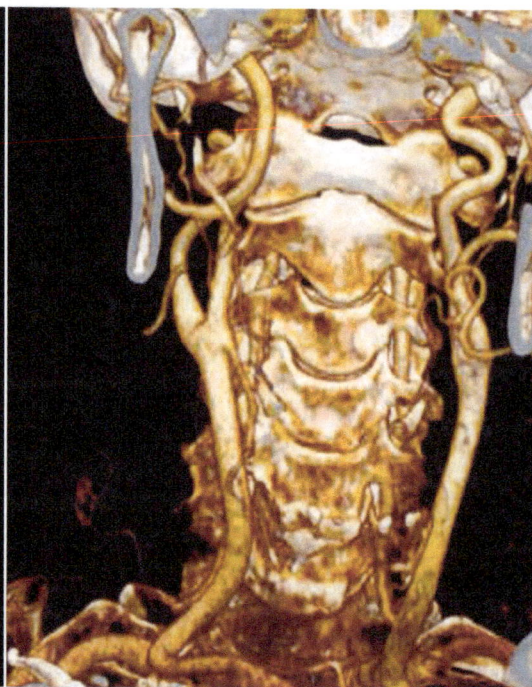

[2] VR of DE bone-unremoved image shows bony structures and carotid arteries at one time.

Findings

With the DE bone removal technique, it was easy to visualize the Willis circle. A significant stenosis at the segment of the right internal carotid of the Willis circle and mild multi-segmental stenosis of the middle cerebral arteries appeared quite satisfying. No abnormalities of the common carotid arteries and the carotid bifurcation were found.

Take-home message

With Dual Energy scanning, the direct subtraction of bone can be achieved almost instantly with a high degree of accuracy. The images of bone removal can cope with the limitation of the complicated skull base, show the abnormalities of the Willis circle clearly and increase the sensitivity in detecting small aneurysms.

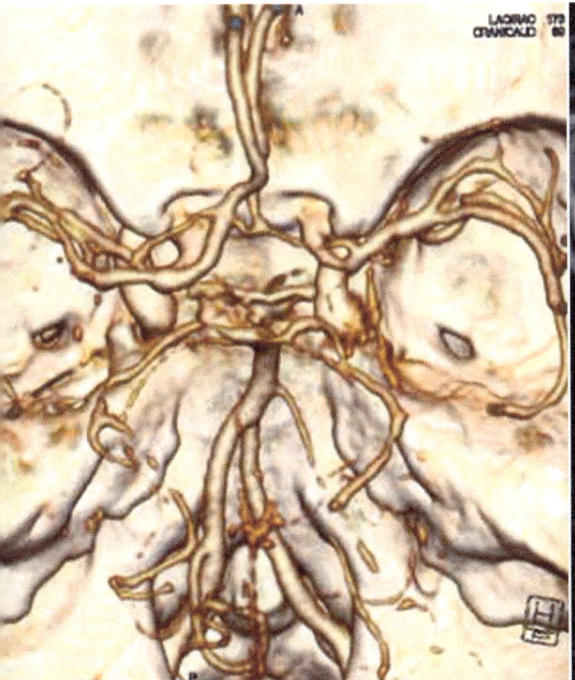

[3] VRT reconstruction mode shows the intracranial vessels.

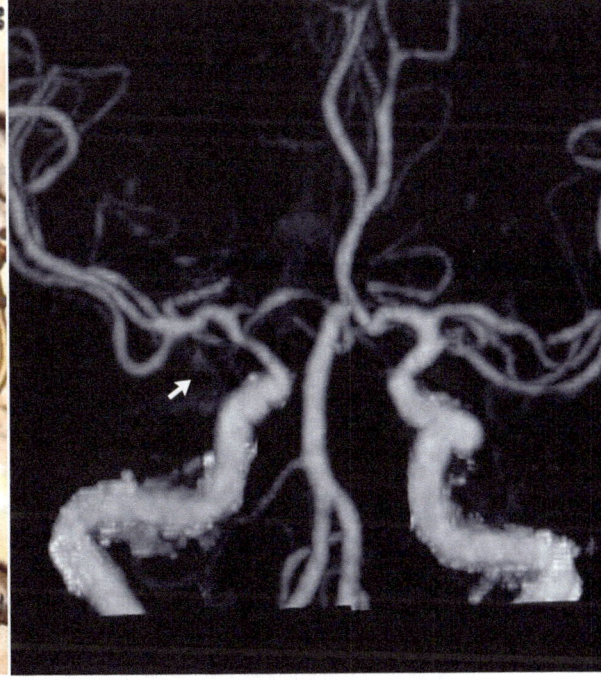

[4] VR image after bone removal displays a significant stenosis (arrow) at the segment of the right internal carotid artery of the Willis circle and mild multi-segmental stenosis of the bilateral middle cerebral arteries.

Dual Energy
CTA Aorta

Li Peiling
Chai Ruimei
Wang Qiang
Xu Ke

Department of Radiology
1st Affiliated Hospital of China Medical University
Shenyang, China

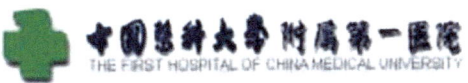
中国医科大学附属第一医院
THE FIRST HOSPITAL OF CHINA MEDICAL UNIVERSITY

Dual Energy
CTA Aorta

Basic considerations

The patient is placed on the table in a supine position. In most cases, the complete aorta from the aortic root to the inguinal arteries should be imaged to be able to rule out aortic dissection, which may extend into the thorax or originate from the thorax. No ECG-gating is necessary for the abdominal aorta. The examination should start with a non-enhanced scan for the whole scan field to be able to rule out intramural haematoma and to allow for differentiation of calcifications from bleeding. The bolus tracking region of interest (ROI) is placed on the descending aorta and the scan is started with a scan delay of seven seconds. [1]

Scan Parameters

Scan mode	Spiral Dual Energy with Dual Source
Scan area	c. trunc to lower limbs *
Scan direction	cranio-caudal
Scan time	~13 s *
Tube voltage A/B	140 kV / 80 kV
Tube current A/B	80 quality ref. mAs / 340 quality ref. mAs *
Dose modulation	CARE Dose4D
$CTDI_{vol}$	~15 mGy *
Rotation time	0.5 s
Pitch	0.65 *
Slice collimation	0.6 mm *
Acquisition	64 x 0.6 mm *
Slice width	2.0 mm *
Reconstruction increment	1.5 mm *
Reconstruction kernel	D30f

* **Asian Adaptation by**
1st Affiliated Hospital of China Medical University
Higher image quality leads to slightly increased values for mAs/rot. and $CTDI_{vol}$.

Tricks

Placing a large bore i.v. line (e.g. 18 G) is essential for optimal bolus administration, which is a prerequisite for high quality CTA, especially with use of DE. For CTA in general, it is not the iodine concentration of the contrast media which is essential but rather the iodine delivery rate (mg I/s) is the main determining factor for optimal enhancement. [1]

Pitfalls

Currently, a non-contrast-enhanced scan is recommended to identify intramural haematoma, and to allow differentiation of calcifications, which may have the appearance of arterial bleeding. A late phase scan is recommended especially after endovascular stent placement to rule out endoleakage. [1]

Contrast Injection Protocol

	Iodine concentration 370 mg I/ml
Injection scheme	Monophasic
Iodine delivery rate	1.48 g/s
CM volume	120 ml
CM flow rate	4 ml/s
Body weight adaptation	no
Bolus timing	bolus tracking **
Bolus tracking threshold	150 HU
ROI position	descending aorta
Scan delay	7 s
Saline flush volume	60 ml
Saline injection rate	4 ml/s
Needle size	18 G
Injection site	antecubital vein

** Depending on the preference of the individual site, test bolus can be used as an alternative

[1] M. Das, A.H. Mahnken, J.E. Wildberger in [1]

Case 1
Suspected Aortic Aneurysm

Case history

A 63-year-old male with sudden severe stomach pain was referred for CT angiography to confirm or rule out aortic aneurysm.

Diagnosis / Differential diagnosis

The aortic CT angiography indicated that the aortic artery and the main branches were all normal. No significant dilatation or stenosis was seen, so the major differential diagnosis for aortic aneurysm was ruled out.

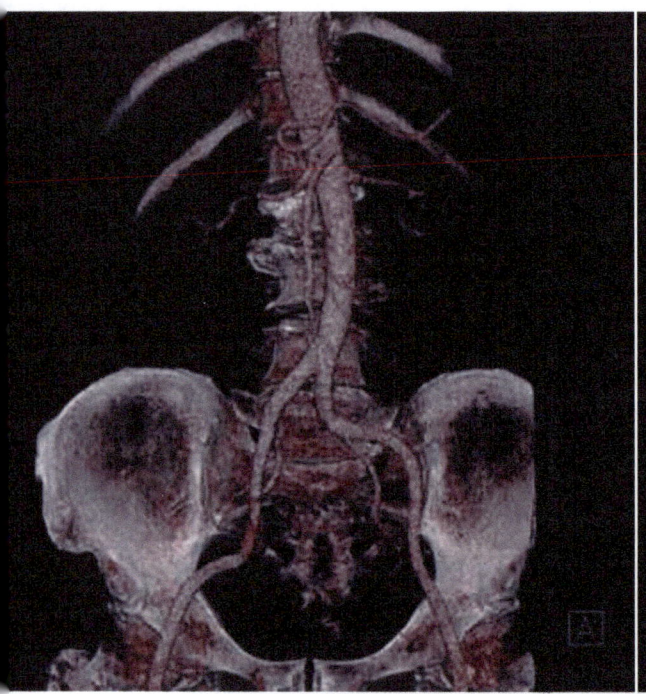

[1] Spiral Dual Energy CTA image of abdomen and pelvis prior to bone subtraction.

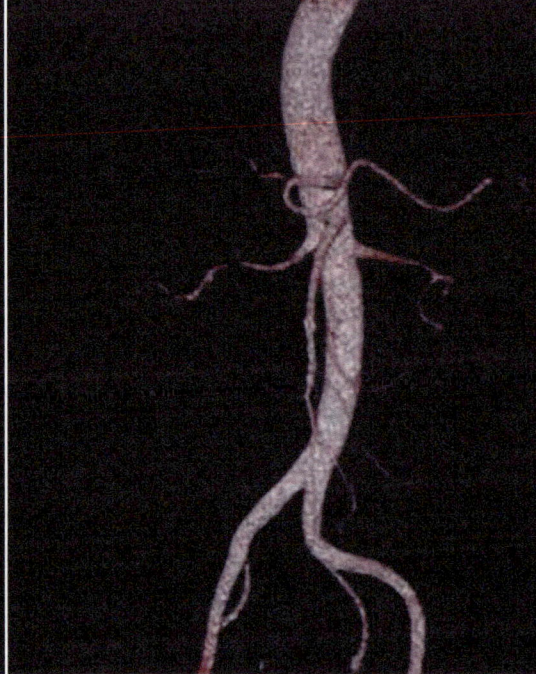

[2] Spiral Dual Energy CTA image of abdomen and pelvis with automatic Dual Energy bone subtraction technique.

Findings

The aortic artery and the main branches had a normal morphology and the respective lumens were unobstructed. No stenosis and no dilatation were seen.

Take-home message

With optimal bolus timing, a high-quality CT angiography of the abdominal aorta is achieved. The use of MPRs allows optimal stent planning. Stent placement shows optimal results eliminating the aneurysm. DSCT is utilized for direct visualization of the aortic aneurysm.

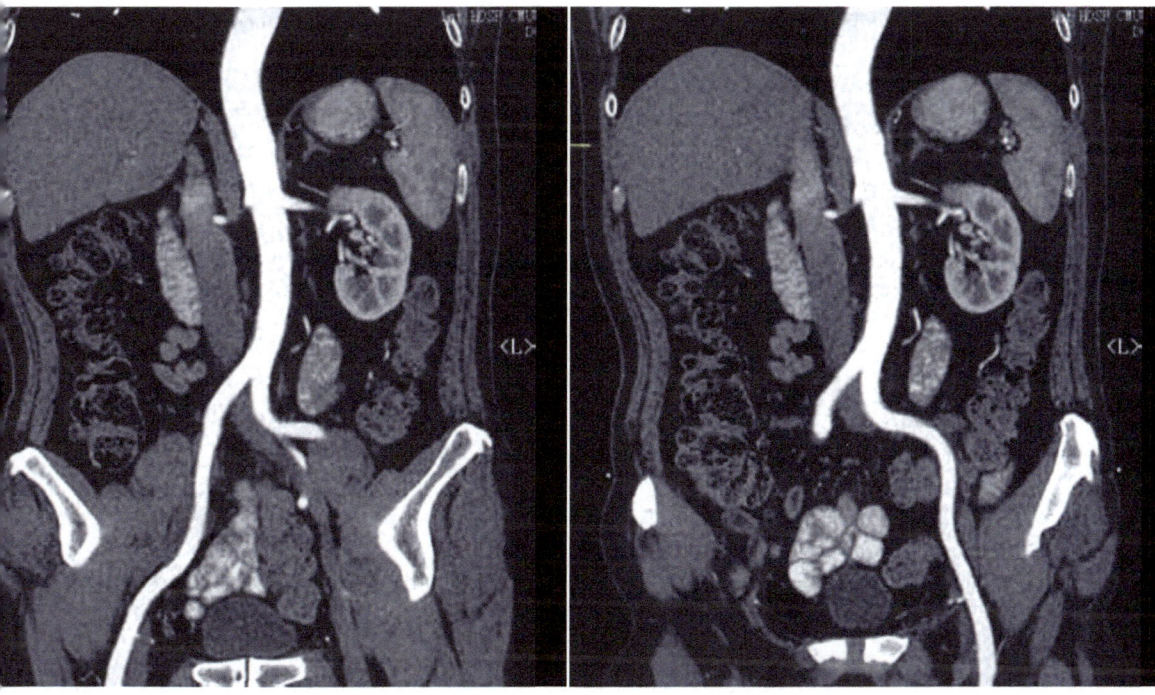

[3] Spiral Dual Energy coronal curved image of abdomen and right common iliac artery.

[4] Spiral Dual Energy coronal curved image of abdomen and left common iliac artery.

Dual Energy
CTA Lung Perfusion (PE)

Eun Jin Chae
Joon Beom Seo
Koun-Sik Song

Department of Radiology and Research Institute of
Radiology
Asan Medical Center
Seoul, Korea

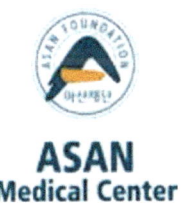

ASAN
Medical Center

Dual Energy
CTA Lung Perfusion (PE)

Basic considerations

Exact positioning of the patient in the isocenter of the gantry is essential to include the peripheral lung in the field of view (FOV). The protocol is aimed at displaying both the pulmonary arteries and pulmonary perfusion. To guarantee sufficient parenchymal enhancement, the scan delay should be longer than for CT angiography. We used a fixed delay of 30 seconds after injection of high concentration contrast agent (370 mg I/ml) followed by a saline chaser.

Scan Parameters

Scan mode	Dual Energy Thorax protocol
Scan area	Thorax*
Scan direction	Caudo-cranial
Scan time	~14 s*
Tube voltage A/B	140 kV/80 kV
Tube current A/B	50/210 effective mAs*
Dose modulation	CARE Dose4D
CTDI$_{vol}$	~12 mGy*
Rotation time	0.33 s
Pitch	0.5*
Slice collimation	1.2 mm
Acquisition	14 x 1.2 mm
Slice width	1.5 mm*
Reconstruction increment	1.0 mm*
Reconstruction kernel	D30f

* **Asian Adaptation by Asan Medical Center**
To assess smaller structures, the resolution is improved by the use of a thinner slice thickness, which results in slightly increased dose values.

Tricks

The scan direction should be caudo-cranial, because dense contrast material will affect the perfusion mapping due to beam hardening. If the scan starts at the diaphragm, the chaser bolus has washed out the superior vena cava by the time the region is scanned. The patient should be instructed to hold his breath at mild inspiration to avoid excessive influx of non-enhanced blood from the inferior vena cava.

Pitfalls

Dense iodine opacification in the superior vena cava and right heart may result in streak artifacts in the lung parenchyma mimicking perfusion defects. To minimize streak artifact, we use the split bolus method including 100% iodine contrast followed by 30% iodine contrast mixed with saline.

Contrast Injection Protocol

	Iodine concentration 370 mg I/ml
Injection scheme	Split bolus method
Iodine delivery rate	1.29 g/s*
CM volume	100 ml*
CM flow rate	3.5 ml/s*
Body weight adaptation	no
Bolus timing	fixed delay*
Bolus tracking threshold	–*
ROI position	–*
Scan delay	30 s (fixed delay)*
Saline flush volume	50 ml (30% contrast + 70% saline)*
Saline injection rate	3.5 ml/s*
Needle size	18 G
Injection site	antecubital vein

Case 1
Acute Pulmonary Embolism

Case history

56-year-old male with leg edema was referred to rule out pulmonary embolism during hospitalization due to brain abscess.

Question

The primary clinical concern was acute pulmonary embolism because he was diagnosed as having deep venous thrombosis and was planned to undergo placement of inferior vena cava (IVC) filter.

Diagnosis / Differential diagnosis

Apart from acute pulmonary embolism, differential diagnoses include right side heart failure, pulmonary hypertension, congestive heart failure, and coronary artery disease.

Findings

Multiple thrombi were found in the right central pulmonary artery, both upper, lower lobar pulmonary arteries, and segmental arteries in

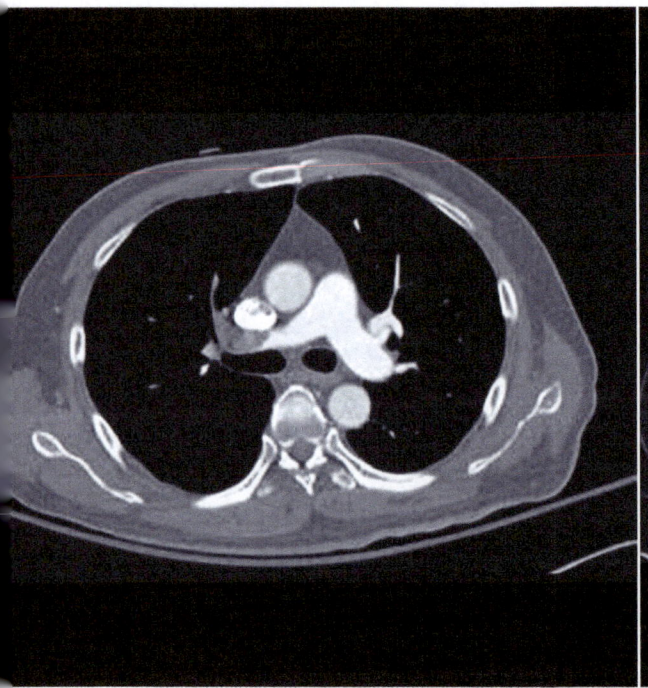 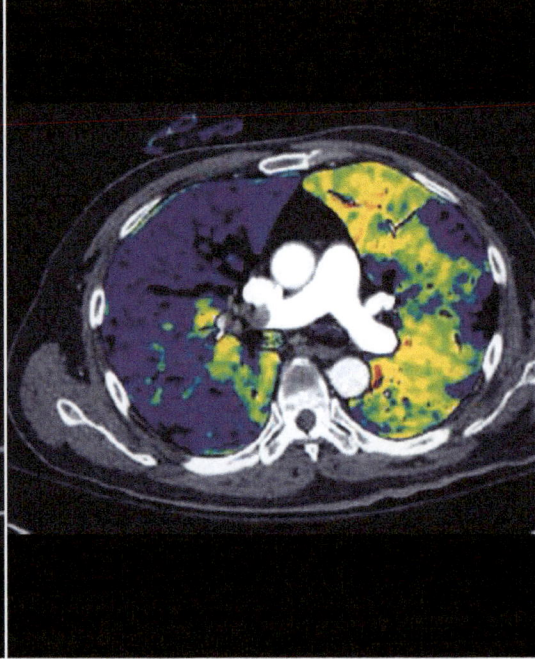

[1] On the axial image of the pulmonary trunk level, there is a large thrombus impacting the right central pulmonary artery.

[2] Perfusion map shows that the perfusion of the right lung profoundly decreases. Additional multifocal perfusion defects are seen in the left lung.

both lungs. On a color-coded perfusion map, multifocal areas of perfusion defect were shown as blue-to-black colored areas and corresponded to the sites of vascular obstruction by thrombi.

Take-home message

Dual Energy CT can show regional perfusion status in the lung in addition to intravascular filling defect in acute pulmonary embolism. This provides a new functional insight into acute pulmonary embolism and makes a more comprehensive assessment possible. Combined assessment of perfusion and vascular obstruction may be used for a better understanding of the severity of and for proper management of patients with pulmonary embolism.

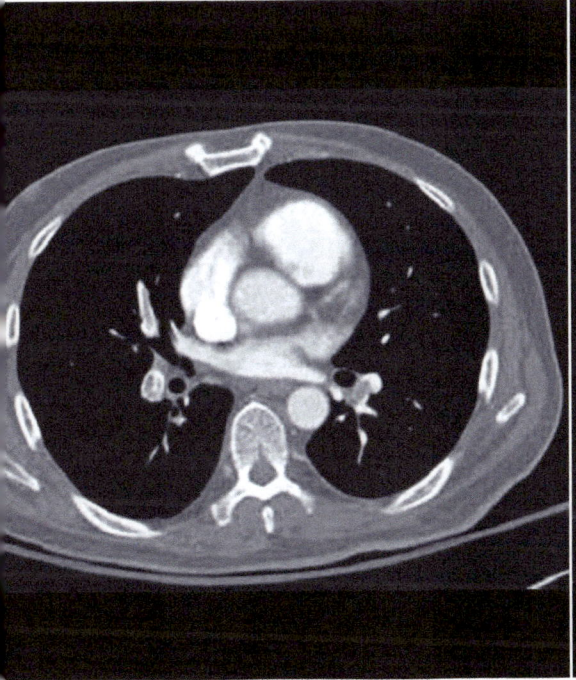 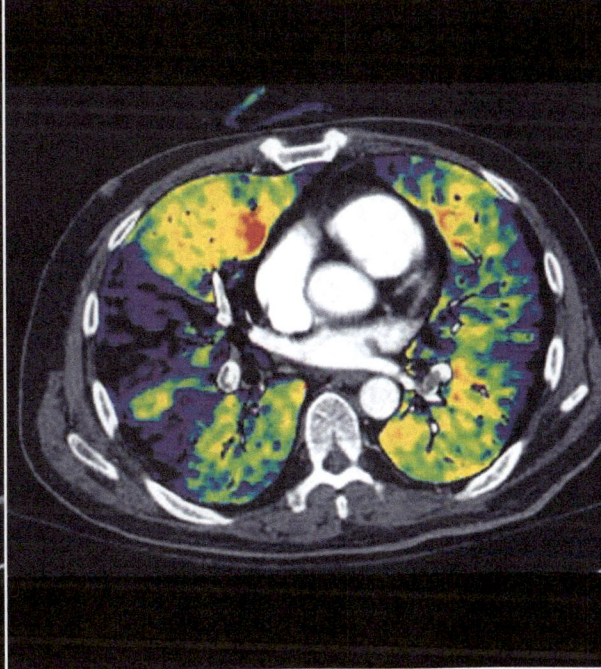

[3] On the axial image of the left inferior pulmonary vein level, there are multiple, small thrombi in the segmental arteries in the right middle and both lower lobes.

[4] On the perfusion map, there are multifocal perfusion defects in both lungs, which are correspondent to the sites of vascular obstruction.

Case 2
Pulmonary Arterial Stenosis/Anthracofibrosis

Case history

73-year-old female with dyspnea and dry cough was referred to rule out acute pulmonary embolism or other lung diseases.

Question

CT angiography was performed not only to rule out pulmonary embolism and but also to investigate the cause of dyspnea.

Diagnosis / Differential diagnosis

Apart from pulmonary embolism, differential diagnoses included pulmonary tuberculosis or pneumonia.

Findings

There was ill-defined soft tissue encircling the right upper lobar bronchus and truncus anterior of the right pulmonary artery. On bronchoscopy, the right upper lobar bronchus showed severe

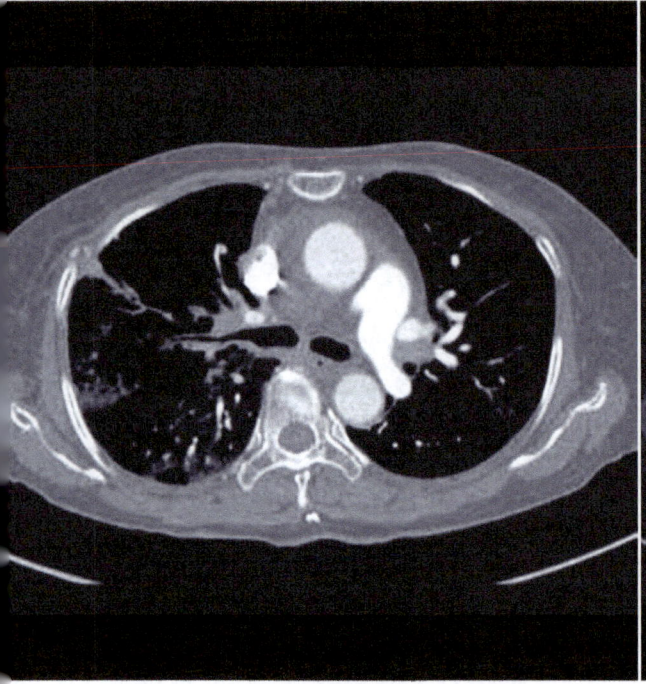 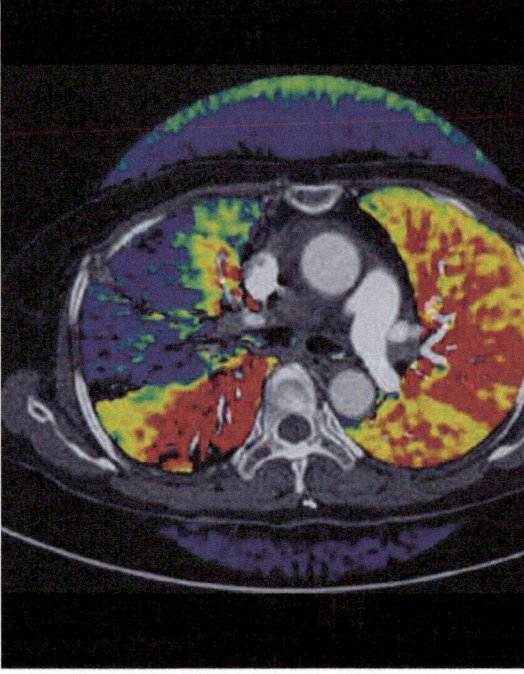

[1] On axial image of the pulmonary trunk level, there is an ill-defined soft tissue encircling the right upper lobar bronchus and truncus anterior of the right pulmonary artery.

[2] Axial perfusion map shows a large perfusion defect probably due to arterial stenosis at the right hilar area.

stenosis and anthracotic pigmentation. On a pathologic specimen obtained by bronchoscopy, there was fibrotic tissue around the right upper lobar bronchus. The patient was diagnosed as having anthracofibrosis according to those findings seen on CT, bronchoscopy and biopsy. It is likely that the patient's dyspnea may be attributable to the large area of decreased perfusion in the right upper lobe, owing to stenosis of the right upper pulmonary artery.

Take-home message

CTA of the thorax using Dual Energy CT simultaneously provides CT angiographic feature and perfusion status by obtaining a color-coded perfusion map. This protocol could be used for various pulmonary vascular diseases such as congenital or acquired pulmonary artery stenosis. We may investigate the cause of pulmonary arterial stenosis and consequent impairment of parenchymal perfusion, allowing more comprehensive understanding of the patient's functional status.

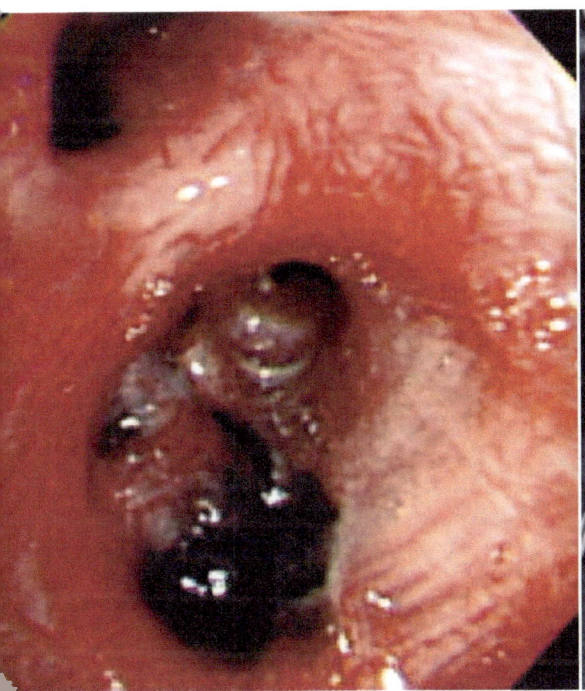

[3] On bronchoscopy, there was a severe stenosis and anthracotic pigmentation in the right upper lobar bronchus, which suggestive of anthracofibrosis.

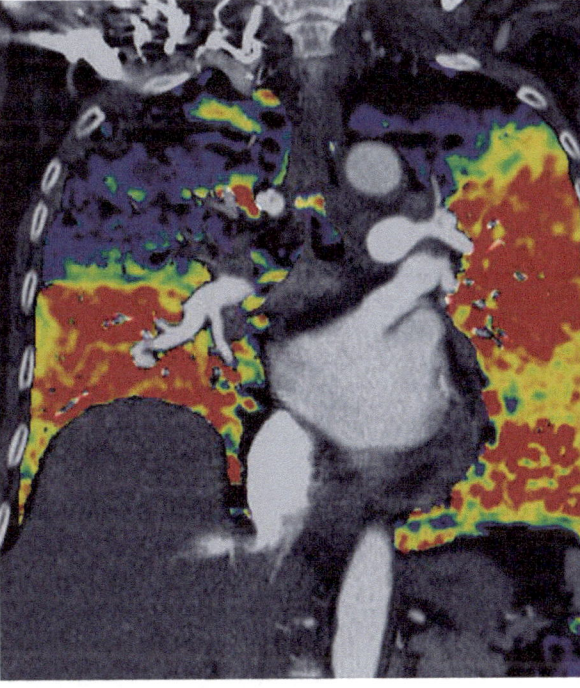

[4] The localized perfusion defect in the right upper lobe is well depicted on coronal perfusion map as well.

Dual Energy
Virtual Non-Contrast

Li Peiling
Chai Ruimei
Wang Qiang
Xu Ke

Department of Radiology
1st Affiliated Hospital of China Medical University
Shenyang, China

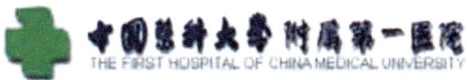
中国医科大学附属第一医院
THE FIRST HOSPITAL OF CHINA MEDICAL UNIVERSITY

Dual Energy
Virtual Non-Contrast

Basic considerations

The virtual non-enhanced imaging protocol is a technique applicable for many indications. Examination of parenchymal organs such as renal scans, liver scans or even vascular scans may require images of non-enhanced phase and thus accumulate radiation dose for any given patient. In most cases, however, the non-enhanced scan does not really contribute to the diagnosis, but it is difficult to predict its necessity in advance. Virtual non-enhanced imaging allows for obtaining non-enhanced scans out of any contrast-enhanced scan at a lower dose when compared with combined scanning protocols.

This holds true for any contrast phase, since the protocol removes iodine from the image while maintaining all underlying structures. [1]

Scan Parameters (exemplified for liver)

Scan mode	Spiral Dual Energy with Dual Source
Scan area	liver/abdomen *
Scan direction	cranio-caudal
Scan time	variable, depending on scan length *
Tube voltage A/B	140 kV / 80 kV
Tube current A/B	95 quality ref. mAs / 404 quality ref. mAs
Dose modulation	CARE Dose4D
$CTDI_{vol}$	~19 mGy
Rotation time	1 s / 0.5 s
Pitch	0.55
Slice collimation	1.2 mm
Acquisition	14 x 1.2 mm
Slice width	1.5 mm
Reconstruction increment	1 mm
Reconstruction kernel	D30s/D30f

* Asian Adaptation by
1st Affiliated Hospital of China Medical University

Tricks

In order to get full scan coverage of the liver, position the patient off-center. For other indications, the patient should be placed in the isocenter. Reduce the rotation time of the gantry to 1 s, if possible. For aortic scans, the rotation time may be 0.5 s. [1]

Pitfalls

The only parameter to consider carefully is the patient's positioning. Problematic combinations are lateral liver segments VI/VII in combination with the left kidney, as not all organs are within the 26 cm field of view in most patients. [1]

Contrast Injection Protocol

	Iodine concentration 370 mg I/ml
Injection scheme	Monophasic
Iodine delivery rate	1.11 g/s – 1.85 g/s
CM volume	80 – 120 ml
CM flow rate	3 – 5 ml/s
Body weight adaptation	no
Bolus timing	–
Bolus tracking threshold	–
ROI position	–
Scan delay	–
Saline flush volume	50 ml
Saline injection rate	3 – 5 ml/s
Needle size	18 G
Injection site	antecubital vein

[1] A. Kuettner, K. Anders, M. Lell in [1]

Case 1
Primary Hepatic Carcinoma

Case history

A 61-year-old female complained of right upper abdominal pain. Ultrasound detected an occupying lesion in the liver.

Diagnosis / Differential diagnosis

The enhanced CT indicated that the lesion in the liver might be a hepatic carcinoma.

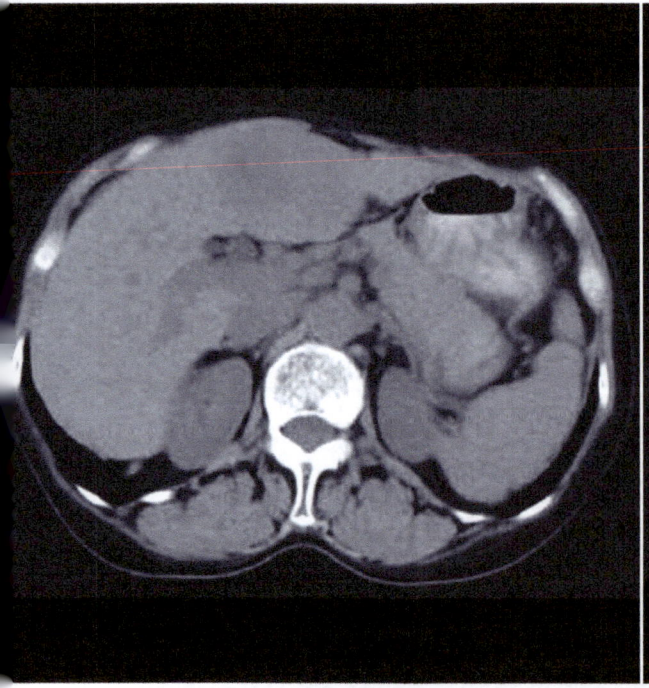

[1] Conventional non-enhanced scan of the liver. The left hepatic lobe showed a low density mass.

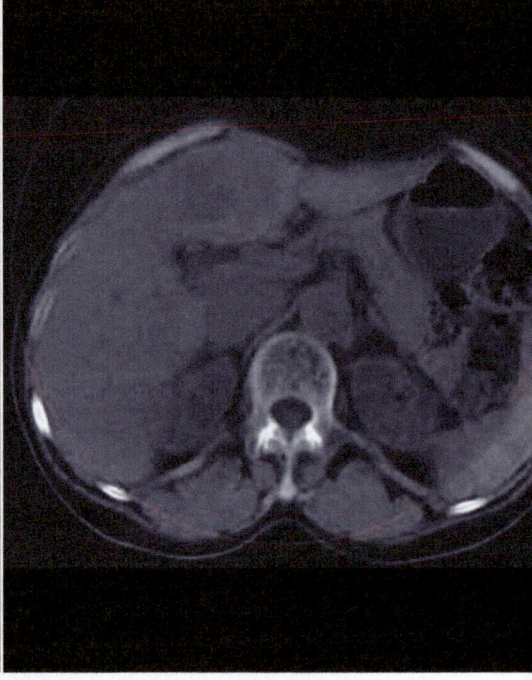

[2] The virtual non-enhanced image could also disclose the lesion clearly, showed no difference from the conventional image.

Findings

The left hepatic lobe was occupied by a large irregular mass with non-uniform enhancement in the atrial phase and portal phase. The left branch of the portal vein was invaded by the mass. These findings made the presence of a primary hepatic carcinoma very likely.

Take-home message

The case demonstrates that the use of Dual Energy scanning may make any non-enhanced scan phase obsolete. The scan technique provides the flexibility to reconstruct a non-enhanced image when needed. But the virtual non-contrast image does not clearly show the margin of lesion. The virtual non-enhanced imaging technique cannot replace routine plain scan completely.

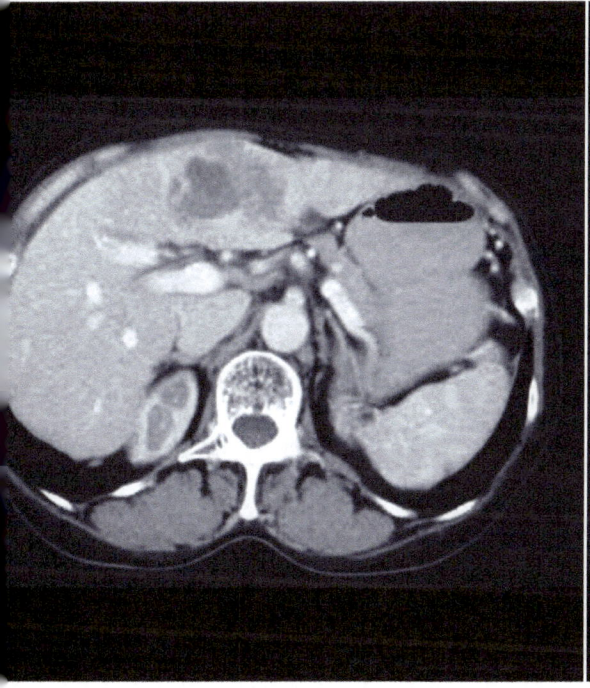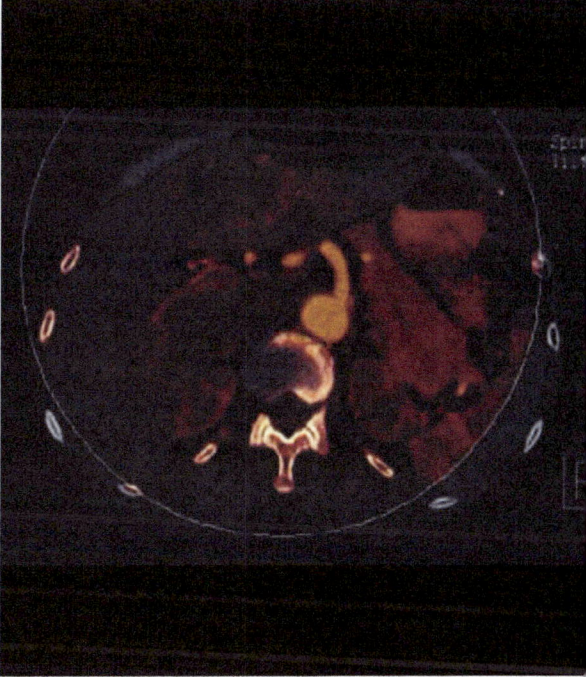

[3] Conventional portal venous phase image. The same slice as image 1. The mass showed irregular enhancement, especially at the peripheral region.

[4] The color-coding image discloses the non-uniform iodine content of the mass.

Case 2
Cholangiocarcinoma

Case history

A 73-year-old female presented with an unclear abdominal pain for 2 months.

Diagnosis / Differential diagnosis

A carcinoma of the gallbladder was accompanied by multi-intrahepatic metastasis and lymphadenectasis.

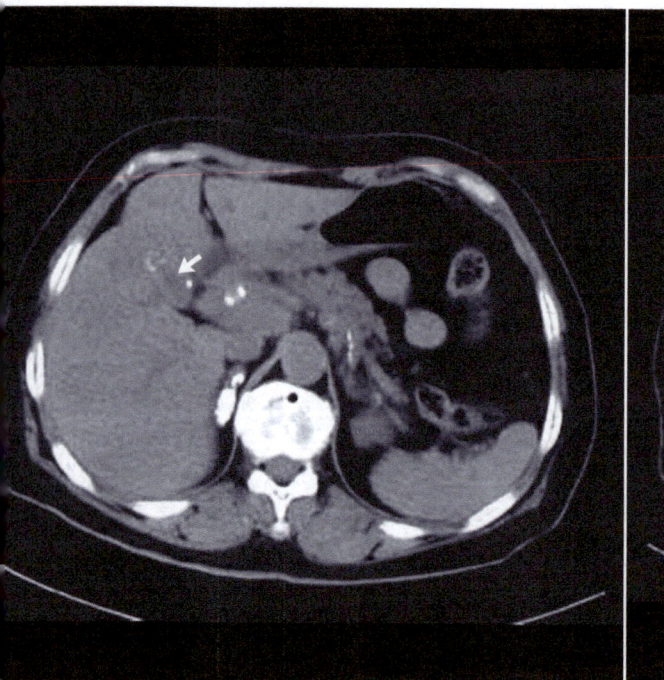

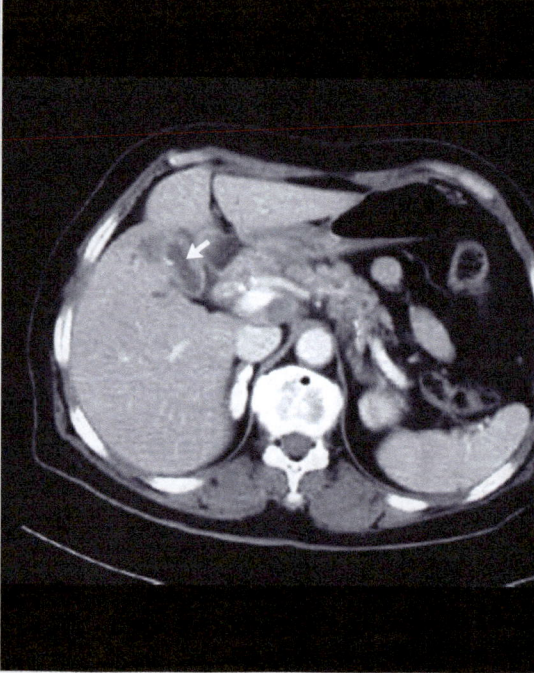

[1] Conventional non-enhanced scan of the liver and gallbladder (arrow). The wall and duct of the gallbladder showed irregular thickening with dotted calcification.

[2] Conventional portal venous scan. Same slice as image 1. Note the apparent contrast enhancement of the wall and duct of gallbladder (arrow).

Findings

The wall and the duct of the gallbladder thickened irregularly, with an unclear margin and a delay enhancement.

The nearby hepatic tissue showed low density. A diagnosis of carcinoma of the gallbladder was suspected and later confirmed by surgery.

Take-home message

The two cases demonstrate that the use of Dual Energy scanning may make any non-enhanced scan phase obsolete. The scan technique gives one the flexibility to reconstruct a non-enhanced image when needed. But the virtual non-contrast image does not clearly show the margin of lesion. The virtual non-enhanced imaging technique cannot replace routine plain scan completely.

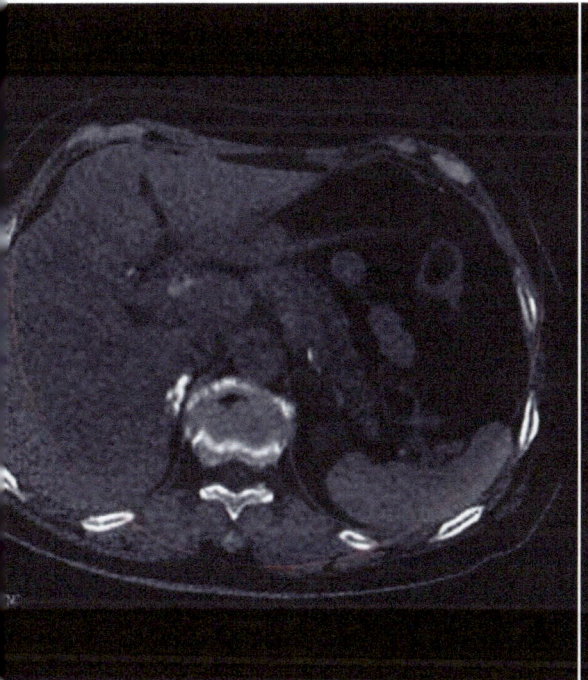 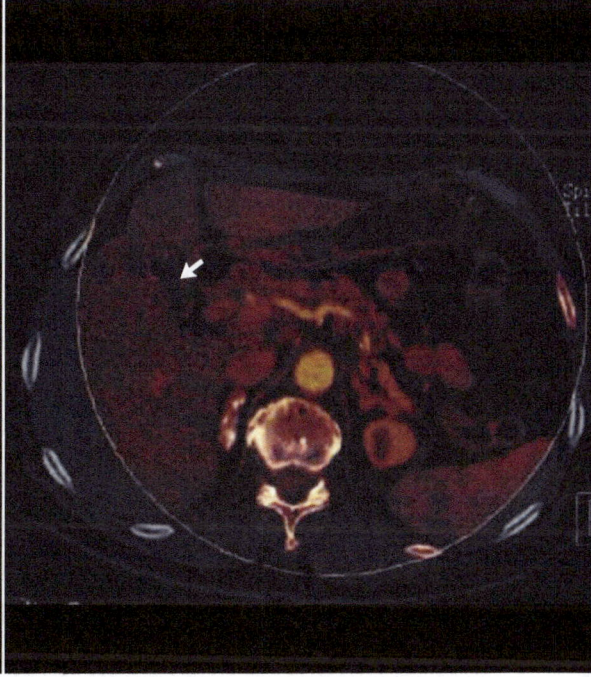

[3] The virtual non-enhanced image is not different from the conventional image.

[4] The color-coding image discloses the iodine content of the gallbladder wall (arrow).

Dual Energy
Vascular Plaque
Detection / Removal

Liu Wei
Xue Huadan
Chen Yu
Sun Hao
Wang Xuan
Jin Zhengyu

Department of Radiology
Peking Union Medical College Hospital
Beijing, China

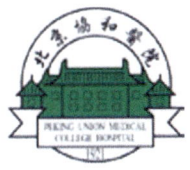

Dual Energy
Vascular Plaque Detection / Removal

Basic considerations

Because Dual Energy plaque detection/removal can be performed in any part of the body, the examination protocol design is variable, depending on the body region examined. Apart from choosing a different scan mode (Dual Energy), the procedure resembles conventional CTA with the iodine delivery rate as the decisive factor determining contrast attenuation.

A $CTDI_{vol}$ comparable to conventional CTA should be delivered. Scan direction should be selected as to achieve an optimal arterial phase, i.e. cranio-caudal for abdomen and caudo-cranial for neck.[1]

Scan Parameters (exemplified for the neck region)

Scan mode	Spiral Dual Energy with Dual Source
Scan area	all supraaortic vessels *
Scan direction	cranio-caudal *
Scan time	~9 s *
Tube voltage A/B	140 kV / 80 kV
Tube current A/B	55 quality ref. mAs / 234 quality ref. mAs
Dose modulation	CARE Dose4D
$CTDI_{vol}$	~10 mGy *
Rotation time	0.33 s *
Pitch	0.7
Slice collimation	0.6 mm
Acquisition	64 x 0.6 mm
Slice width	0.75 mm *
Reconstruction increment	0.5 mm *
Reconstruction kernel	D20f *

* **Asian Adaptation by PUMC, Beijing**
Since the patient population in Asia is typically slimmer than in the US and Europe, faster rotation times can be used without reaching the system limits.

Tricks

Tube current modulation (CARE Dose4D) should be switched on to smooth the image noise profile of the scan for an efficient Dual Energy analysis. Scanning should be performed in an early arterial phase. [1]

Pitfalls

Spiral Dual Energy evaluation is only possible within the inner field of view of 26 cm in the center of the gantry, therefore the patient has to be positioned carefully. In obese patients or in anatomical regions with irregular attenuation profiles such as the shoulders, image quality might be degraded if scan parameters are not adjusted accordingly. [1]

Contrast Injection Protocol

	Iodine concentration 370 mg I/ml
Injection scheme	Monophasic
Iodine delivery rate	1.85 g/s
CM volume	80 ml
CM flow rate	5 ml/s
Body weight adaptation	no
Bolus timing	bolus tracking **
Bolus tracking threshold	130 HU
ROI position	aortic arch
Scan delay	2 s
Saline flush volume	60 ml
Saline injection rate	5 ml/s
Needle size	18 G
Injection site	antecubital vein

** Depending on the preference of the individual site, test bolus can be used as an alternative

[1] C. Thomas, H. Brodoefel, M. Heuschmid, A. Kopp in [1]

Case 1
Mild Calcification of the Carotid Artery

Case history

A 59-year-old male complained of onset of dizziness and vomiting. The patient had a long history of hypertension, hyperlipidemia, coronary artery disease and long-term smoking. There was no history of stroke or transient ischemic attack.

Diagnosis / Differential diagnosis

Atherosclerotic changes of the supraaortic vessels with multiple bilateral stenosis of the common carotid arteries (CCAs) and internal carotid arteries (ICAs) were detected.

Findings

Atherosclerotic changes of the bilateral carotid arteries were found. There was severe stenosis of the proximal part of the right ICA and middle-grade stenosis of the siphon part of the left ICA. Selective Dual-Energy-based bone removal offered excellent motion-artifact-free results but

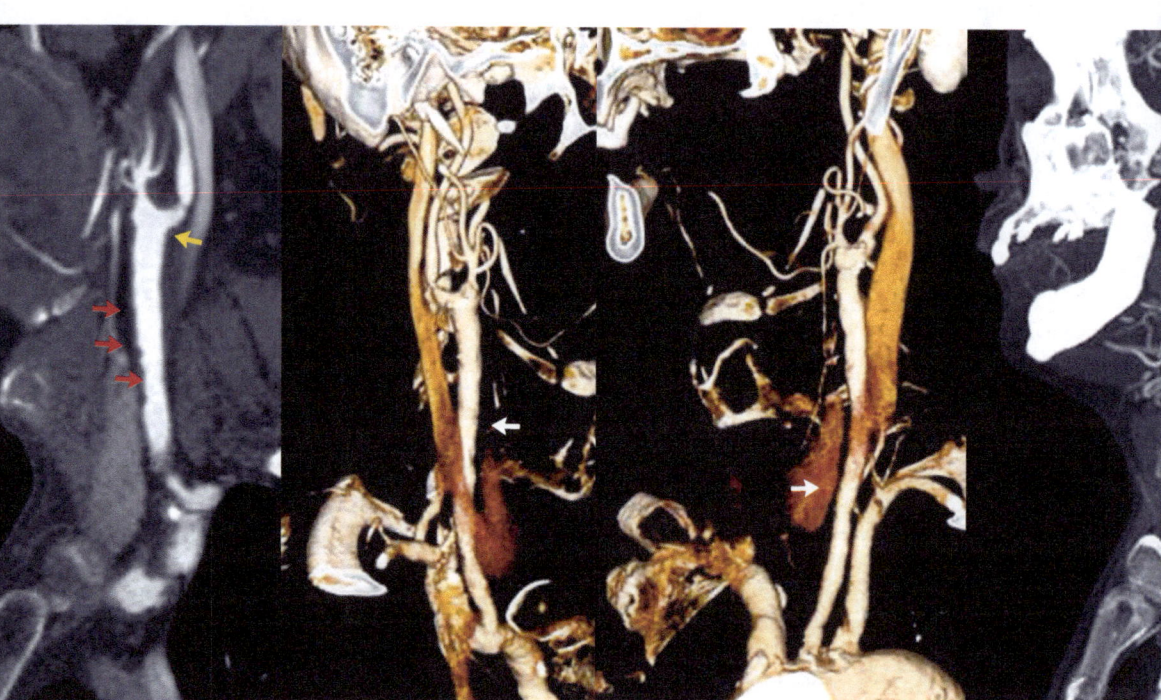

[1] MPR demonstrates multiple plaques with lipid contents (red arrows) of the right common carotid artery (CCA) and high-grade stenosis (yellow arrow) of the internal carotid artery (ICA).

VRT and MIP images demonstrate the bilateral CCAs and the internal carotid arteries below the skull base. Note the multiple plaques and irregularities of the bilateral common carotid arteries (grey arrows).

remnants of the calcified plaque were noted. The enhancement of the cavernous sinus somewhat obscured the siphon segment of the ICA.

Take-home message

Dual Energy CTA (DE-CTA) demonstrates excellent bone subtraction ability. It can display the whole range of extra- and intra-cranial arteries. With Dual-Energy-based bone removal, postprocessing of carotid CTA may be easier and less user-dependent. With technique improvement, the margin of vessel after bone subtraction becomes more and more smooth, which increases the diagnostic confidence. In the case of patients with suspicion of stenosis of intracranial arteries, a cranio-caudal scan direction is preferred to avoid venous contamination.

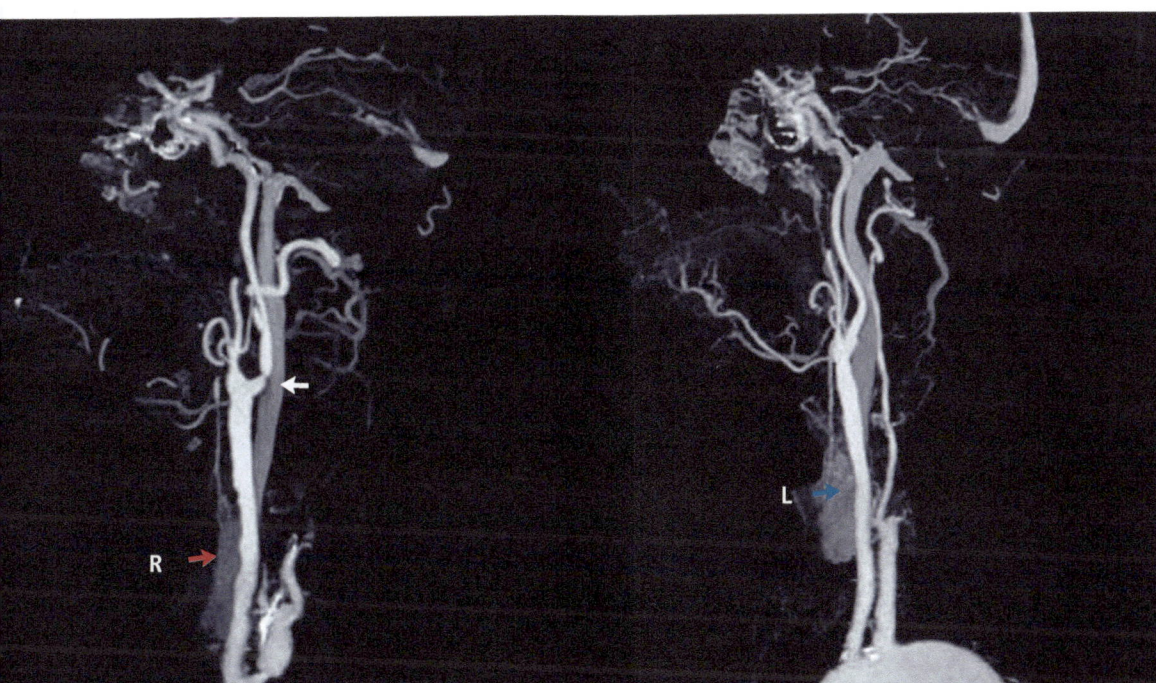

[2] DECT bone removal images display the whole range of bilateral carotid arteries (CA) and vertebral arteries (VA). Note multiple calcification (red arrow) of the siphon part of the right internal carotid artery (ICA) and irregularity of the bilateral common carotid arteries (blue arrow). There is high-grade stenosis (white arrow) of the proximal part of the right internal carotid artery (ICA).

Case 2
Severe Calcification of the Carotid Artery

Case history

A 57-year-old female presented with mild left-sided weakness. She had a long history of hypertension. Multiple small ischemic lesions at the right hemisphere were seen on a non-enhanced CT scan of the head.

Diagnosis/Differential diagnosis

Atherosclerotic changes of the bilateral carotid arteries were observed. Calcified plaque of the bilateral carotid bifurcation could be seen. There was moderate stenosis of the proximal part of the right ICA due to the mixed-content plaque.

Findings

Dual Energy images showed calcified plaques at both carotid bifurcations. Dual-Energy-based bone removal offered excellent motion-artifact-free results. Moderate stenosis of the right internal carotid artery was detected due to

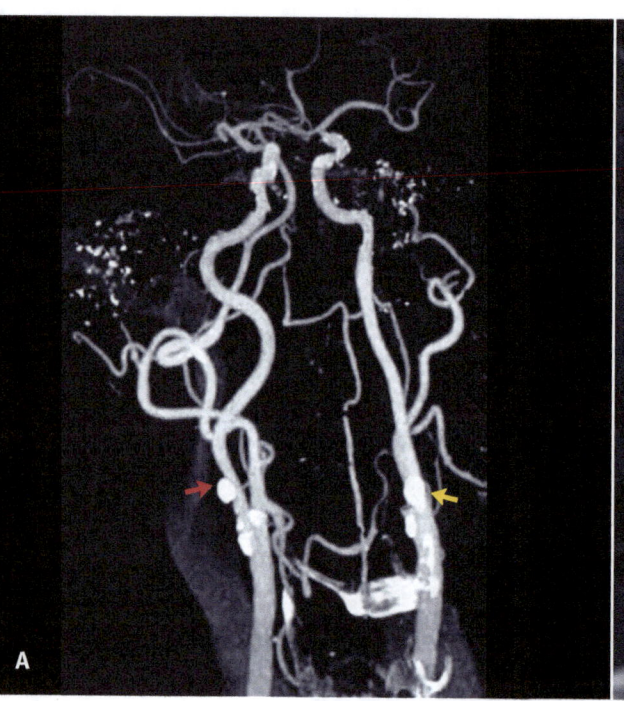 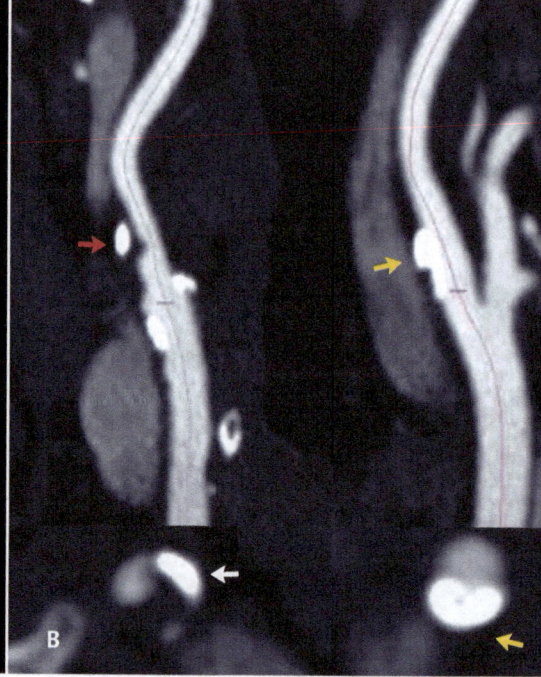

A. Plaque on: Calcified plaques at both carotid bifurcations. Plaque on the right internal carotid artery (ICA) contains lipid content (white arrow in Figure B).

B. Axial and CPR images: Moderate stenosis of the right ICA is detected due to calcified and soft plaque (red arrows in Figures A, B, C).

calcified and soft plaque. Severe vascular stenosis was not found in the left carotid artery.

Take-home message

With modified scan protocols, the intracranial arteries display with less venous contamination. Dual Energy CTA enables a differentiation of iodine-filled vessel lumina from calcified vessel plaques, making a more accurate quantification of carotid stenosis possible. By using the Dual Energy bone removal tool, plaque with lipid content can be removed with a smooth margin. Calcified plaque near the vessel lumen can exaggerate the stenosis grading due to the irregular margin, or be removed with remnants. Further investigations and comparison with DSA need to be done for accuracy evaluation.

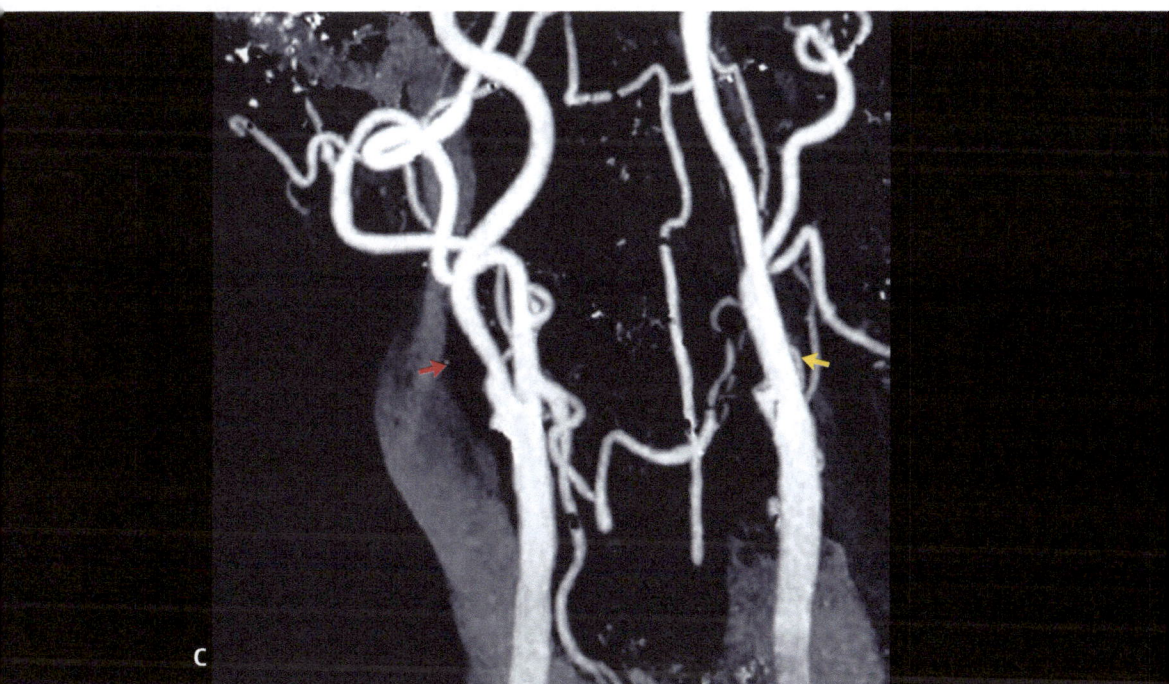

C. Plaque off: Severe vascular stenosis was not found in the left carotid artery (yellow arrows in Figures A, B, C).

Abbreviations

AAA	abdominal aortic aneurysm		LVOT	left ventricular outflow tract
AF	atrial fibrillation		MB	myocardial bridging
ASD	atrial septal defect		MCA	middle cerebral artery
BMI	body mass index		MDCT	multi-detector row CT
bpm	beats per minute		MI	myocardial infarction
CABG	cardiac/coronary artery bypass graft		MIP	maximum intensity projection
CAD	coronary artery disease		MPR	multiplanar reformation
CBF	cerebral blood flow		MRA	magnetic resonance angiography
CBV	cerebral blood volume		MRI	magnetic resonance imaging
CCA	common carotid artery		MSCT	multislice spiral CT
CCTA	coronary CT angiography		MTT	mean transit time
CKMB	creatine kinase myocardial band		NECT	non-enhanced CT
CM	contrast media		OM	obtuse marginal branch
CNR	contrast-to-noise ratio		p.a.	posteroanterior
CPR	curved planar reformation		PAOD	peripheral arterial occlusive disease
CRT	cardiac resynchronization therapy		PBV	perfused blood volume
CT	computed tomography		PCI	percutaneous coronary intervention
CTA	CT angiography		PCT	perfusion CT
CTDIvol	computed tomography dose index		PDA	posterior descending artery
CTO	total coronary artery occlusion		PE	pulmonary embolism
CTP	CT perfusion (scan)		RAS	renal artery stenosis
CTU	CT urography		RCA	right coronary artery
CX	circumflex artery		RCC	renal cell carcinoma
DECT	Dual Energy CT		RCX	right circumflex artery
DSA	digital subtraction angiography		RFCA	radio-frequency catheter ablation
DSCT	Dual Source CT		ROA	regurgitant orifice area
DWI	diffusion-weighted imaging		ROI	region of interest
EBCT	electron beam CT		R-R interval	time between two successive R-waves
ECG	electrocardiogram			resp. heart beats
ECHO	echocardiogram		RVOT	right-ventricular outflow tract
EDV	end-diastolic volume		SAH	subarachnoid hemorrhage
EF	ejection fraction		SNR	signal-to-noise ratio
ESV	end-systolic volume		SPECT	single-photon emission CT
EVAR	endovascular aortic repair		SSD	shaded surface display
FMD	fibromuscular dysplasia		s/p	status post
FoV	field of view		SVC	superior vena cava
Gd-DTPA	gadolinium diethylene triaminopentaacetic acid		SVG	scalable vector graphics
			T_{rot}	rotation time
HU	Hounsfield units		TTP	time-to-peak
ICA	internal carotid artery		VE	virtual endoscopy
ICD	implantable cardioverter defibrillator		VRT	volume-rendering technique
IMA	internal mammary arteries		VSD	ventricular septal defect
IVC	inferior vena cava			
IVUS	intravascular ultrasound			
LAD	left anterior descending artery			
LCX	left circumflex artery			
LVH	left-ventricular hypertrophy			

Batch number: 09417118

Printed by Printforce, the Netherlands